For Sam and Rhoda

PRAISE FOR BRIAN FRAZER'S
HYPER-CHONDRIAC

"Hilarious and biting . . . wickedly funny observation[s]."
—*Entertainment Weekly*

"A riotous romp through a head case's attempts to find inner peace for his own bodily health."
—*New York Post*

"How did Brian Frazer take his neuroses and write a hysterical book, while mine just annoy my family? Seriously, this is one funny book. Damn it."
—Ray Romano

"*Hyper-chondriac* is my new favorite memoir! It was so funny I laughed out loud, so honest I gasped out loud and so relatable I immediately called my therapist. I love this book!"
—Stefanie Wilder-Taylor, author of
Sippy Cups Are Not for Chardonnay

"Brian Frazer has written a very touching and hilarious exploration of family, hypochondria and road rage. It's awesome."
—Greg Behrendt, coauthor of
He's Just Not That Into You

HYPER-CHONDRIAC

ONE MAN'S QUEST
TO HURRY UP
AND CALM DOWN

BRIAN FRAZER

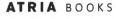

ATRIA BOOKS

NEW YORK LONDON
TORONTO SYDNEY

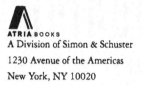
ATRIA BOOKS
A Division of Simon & Schuster
1230 Avenue of the Americas
New York, NY 10020

First Atria Books trade paperback edition March 2008

ATRIA BOOKS and colophon are trademarks of Simon & Schuster, Inc.

For information about special discounts for bulk purchases,
please contact Simon & Schuster Special Sales at
1-800-456-6798 or business@simonandschuster.com.

Manufactured in the United States of America

10 9 8 7 6 5 4 3 2 1

The Library of Congress has cataloged the hardcover edition as follows:
Frazer, Brian.
    Hyper-chondriac : one man's quest to hurry up and calm down / Brian Frazer.
        p.   cm.
        1. Frazer, Brian—Health. 2. Hypochondria—Patients—Biography. 3. Medicine,
Psychosomatic. I. Title.
    RC552.H8F73 2007
    362.196'85250092—dc22   2006052131
    ISBN-13: 978-0-7432-9339-6

ISBN-13: 978-0-7432-9342-6 (pbk)

CONTENTS

Everything in this book is true. However, some names were changed to protect the innocent. Then I realized that I might have changed the names to people I've never met before and I don't want to insult strangers. So I promptly changed them back to people I knew. Sorry for wasting your time with this page. You can rip it out now, if you'd like.

Okay, my lawyers just said that I *do* have to change the names after all. But not mine. Sorry again for the delay in getting to the actual book.

hy·per-chon·dri·a *n.*

The frenetic combustion in one's brain that creates external and internal disease and makes one very unpleasant company to family, peers, the medical community and even oneself.

INTRODUCTION

ITCHING

My hands were itching. After scratching my palms furiously for about an hour, they were still itching, so I drove to the pharmacy and spent thirty bucks on creams, lotions and gels. The trip was a quick one since I knew the exact aisle and shelf of every cream, lotion and gel (and capsule and tablet and cough expectorant). An hour later, my cream/lotion/gel–coated hands continued to itch, so I called a friend. Josh had been living in Los Angeles longer than I and seemed privy to every local specialist, whereas my collection of doctors was scattered between Boston, New York and Southern California. He referred me to his dermatologist, Dr. Tamm.

Dr. Tamm was a stern, bespectacled man of about sixty. He also wore what appeared to be a welder's mask over his thick glasses, apparently so he could see so deeply into peoples' pores that he could make eye contact with the gray matter in their brains.

Here's what I expected to happen in that office visit.

"Hi, my hands itch."

"Use some of this, son!" Dr. Tamm would reply while removing a tube of extra-strength, prescription-only cortisone cream from his front pocket and tossing it to me.

"Thank you, sir! I will."

"See Donna on the way out for your billing information."

This is what actually happened.

"Hi, my hands itch."

"You seem pretty tense."

"Actually, I feel pretty relaxed right now."

"Anything stressful happening in your life at the moment? Did you start a new job? Move? Anything?"

"Well, I'm getting married in a month."

"Are you nervous about the wedding?"

"Not at all. I knew ten minutes into our first date I was going to marry her."

"Congratulations."

"Thanks."

"How'd you meet?"

"Writing thought-bubbles on a TV show called *Blind Date*."

"Never seen it."

"It's like a live comic strip with horny people. I doubt you'd like it."

"So, I don't think your itching has anything to do with the wedding. Or anything else that's going on in your external surroundings."

"You know that already? You've spent like forty-five seconds with me."

"I know, but your energy is overpowering. You're the most uptight, high-strung person I've ever met. The problem isn't in your hands. It's in your head."

Dr. Tamm probably had a point.

On paper I'm the world's healthiest guy. I eat right, exercise regularly, drink in moderation, have all of the good cholesterol and none of the bad, weigh the same as I did in high school, have ideal blood pressure, am caffeine-free, get plenty of sleep, never smoke and have only missed one day of flossing in the last five years. It's essential that I take tip-top care of myself. Because underneath the wholesome habits and exemplary bodily statistics, I'm an unmitigated, non-synergetic mess.

But my body isn't to blame; it's my mind's fault. I've been attempting to regulate this high-maintenance brain of mine since my first baby aspirin. Some kids had guidance counselors. I had hypnotists. Others cried when they got braces. I had anxiety attacks whenever I saw baked beans. Friends collected baseball cards. I collected doctors' cards. Life just didn't feel right unless something was wrong.

For me there's always been a certain calmness in being in the diagnostic chair; then at least there's a reason for why life isn't as satisfying and perfect as I'd like it to be. Although I usually don't know what I've got until the experts tell me, once they do, I'm psyched—as long as there are pills to swallow, creams to rub and warnings to heed. I'm fully capable of generating a new disease every month. Colitis. Prostatitis. Bronchitis (three times, including one stint on antibiotics in England for fifty-seven consecutive days). Hepatitis (the kind that turns you yellow, not the kind that Tommy Lee gave Pamela Anderson). Bigarexia (yes, there is such a thing). And as soon as I've conquered the ailment du jour, I'll just move on to the next disorder. Hastily. But it took a dermatologist to help me realize that I didn't actually have a collection of diseases—I had just one. Hyper-chondria. A word I've made up for my condition.

Now, before I go any further, let me explain the difference between a *hypo*chondriac (not me) and a *hyper*-chondriac (me). Hypochondria is when you think you're sick but you're really not. The hypochondriac's imaginary symptoms and ailments could theoretically be cured with a variety of placebos—be they Halloween candy, dog kibble or a plastic button from a rugby shirt.

Conversely, placebos don't help hyper-chondriacs because hyper-chondriacs actually are sick. Unlike my *hypo* brethren, when I go to the doctor, I think I have ailment X and I do. The seed of each disease originates in my hyper brain, which subsequently creates a swirl of inner turmoil and turbulence in my body.[1]

---

1. In 2005 a group of Australian scientists from the Garvan Institute in Sydney discovered that a hormone released into the body during times of stress, neuropeptide Y (NPY), destabilizes the body's immune system, which makes one susceptible to illness. Don't worry, there won't be many of these. I hate this tiny font as much as you do.

I've always been in a rush to do things: I paced in my crib, I barked at my parents to stir my chocolate milk faster, I ran out my walks in Little League. I would also seek revenge on anyone who impeded my path to getting things done quickly. Seemingly every day of my life I've had to restrain myself from punching people in the face. Before I discovered my hyperchondria, I couldn't even drive more than a mile without honking at someone. And I don't just mean a little tap that says, "Hey . . . um . . . excuse me . . . but the light just changed." I'm talking about holding down the horn with my forehead while simultaneously giving the other car the finger with both hands. Not only was I rushing through life, I was rushing through life in a combative rage. For the better part of my thirty-eight years, my head felt as if it was inhabited by a pair of destructive heavy-metal bands each occupying a brain hemisphere. And neither of them liked the other.

So when Dr. Tamm had a solution to my itchy palms I was ready for action. He pulled out his free drug company pen with the word "Doxycycline" printed on the side and scribbled something on his pad, then tore the page off and stared at me as I read it aloud.

"Zoloft?"

"I think it'll help."

"Isn't that for depression? Because I'm not depressed. It's one of the few things that doesn't seem to happen to me."

"It can be for depression, but it's also used as an anti-anxiety medication."

He proceeded to tell me that Zoloft was a selective serotonin reuptake inhibitor that would help take some of my edge off. Had my friends and family been in the examination room, Dr. Tamm would have undoubtedly been the first dermatologist in history to get a standing ovation.

I needed a wake-up call and it didn't have to be from God or a family intervention or a fellow road-rager teaching me a lesson by shooting me with his assault weapon. Besides, I'd seen those enticing TV commercials for Zoloft where that adorable little circle-creature turns his life around and it looked really appealing. I mean, it totally worked for that little circle-creature.

"Now, there could be side effects such as erection problems, but you let me know if that happens," warned Dr. Tamm.

"Sure."

"And I don't want you to discuss today's treatment with anyone. Don't tell your friends, don't tell your family members, don't even tell your fiancée."

"Why not?"

"It's better if you're not self-conscious about people knowing."

Keeping secrets from my soon-to-be spouse didn't seem like a good way to start a life together. But Dr. Tamm had seen through me in under a minute, so I figured why not let him push the boundaries of his skin doctor degree. Besides, I was sure my fiancée wouldn't have minded. It's not like Nancy wasn't aware she was about to wed a ragey, sick guy.

The first time Nancy slept over she awoke to me stuffing baby diaper rash ointment into each nostril with a Q-tip— a treatment resulting from three months of mind-numbing dizziness in 1995. Two surgeons were convinced I had a brain tumor; thankfully, a third diagnosed it as nasal polyps. I still required an operation, but not the kind where they cut your skull in half like a cantaloupe.

Then there was the Thanksgiving I flew back east to meet Nancy's mother for the first time. In the middle of dinner I politely asked, "Could you please pass the cranber—AUGHHH-HHHHHHHHHHHHHHHHHHHH!!!!!!!!!" I then dropped my silverware on the floor and my head on the table and began frantically massaging my left eyelid. It felt as if someone was stabbing my cornea with an ice pick.

This was due to an accident in 1992 with a newspaper. As I frenetically turned to the sports section of *The Boston Globe*, speed-reading each page in a mad rush to check box scores to find out how my fantasy baseball players did, I flipped one of the corners into the center of my left eye. If you think a paper cut on your thumb hurts, try getting one near your optic nerve.

The eye guy in the emergency room said that I'd scratched my cornea. I was given an eye patch and told to rest both eyes for the next seventy-two hours. As I sat in my dark bedroom, I remember being happy thinking that my life was technically getting a little better since every minute—every second, in fact—my eye was allegedly repairing itself. As much as the hyper-chondriac likes to rush, waiting to heal is equally satisfying. During the follow-up visit, the patch was removed and I was given special drops to put into my eye should the shooting pains return. And if I didn't have the drops, I was told to massage my closed lid for twenty minutes—which Nancy's mom was about to witness on our first Thanksgiving together.

Then there were my numerous colon checkups and blood tests, my bouts with vertigo, the time I required oxygen on a flight back from New York, and the Fourth of July my left arm went numb. Point being, Nancy was accustomed to seeing me at less than full strength. She understood my ailments; perhaps because a thirty-two-ounce bottle of Arizona Iced Tea once slipped out of her cart at Trader Joe's and landed on her foot, causing her to faint. And there was the time she had red spots on her ankles and went to the doctor thinking it was Kaposi's sarcoma. It turned out to be flea bites from her friend's cat. Sometimes I think the only reason Nancy married me is to feel normal in comparison.

I waited at the pharmacy for my Zoloft prescription for nearly an hour. How long does it take to throw thirty pills into a bottle with a cotton ball? The place was empty and I was the only customer! This was bullshit. Hurry up! I'm just one serotonin-not-being-blocked away from snapping! After ten minutes of glaring at the pharmacist, I sat down in the waiting area and watched MSNBC on the ancient RCA that's supposed to make not-being-helped entertaining. They were doing a story about a giant tortoise named Harriet who was collected by Charles Darwin in 1835, and was about to celebrate her 172nd birthday. Harriet had lived through the Civil War, Van Gogh shooting himself, the Panama Canal construction, Prohibition, Jackie Robinson's Major League debut, the moon landing and the final episode of *Friends*. As I watched stock footage of the oldest living animal in the world, I couldn't help noticing that she was moving really, really slowly. Maybe that's why she *was* the oldest living animal in the world. You don't hear about cheetahs or baboons living even a fraction of that. They're way too hyper. It hit me that all animals who have long life spans have one thing in common: they take their time. I mean, elephants may appear to be grossly overweight, but they don't rush and they can live to be seventy. And camels, cool and composed, can easily live to fifty. On the other hand, kangaroos are bouncing off the walls all day. Average life expectancy: nine. I had to be less like a marsupial and more like Harriet. In a scant forty-five minutes, my Zoloft was ready.

But on the way home, I thought the hell with Harriet and started having doubts about being a Zoloftian. I'd always believed that people who were on prescription medication were taking the easy way out. They wanted a quick fix. They were lazy. Weak. They weren't really interested in digging deeper and solving their ills; they just wanted to throw a drop cloth over them. They wanted magic. On the other hand, since our new insurance graciously charged ten bucks for a month's supply of drugs, if I threw them all away, I'd only be out the equivalent of a large tube of Neosporin.

I sat in my kitchen looking at the bottle. After about five minutes of staring, I summoned up the courage to remove the childproof cap, exposing two and a half dozen little blue pills—each of which actually had the word "Zoloft" embossed on it. Which made me even more paranoid. What if you were at a restaurant and you pulled one of them out and someone asked, "What's that?" And you lied and said, "A vitamin." And then this person asked, "What vitamin is blue?" And you'd answer, "Vitamin B . . . that's what the B stands for, y'know, 'blue.'" Meanwhile, the guy sitting on the other side of you has been looking over your shoulder with his laser-corrected eyes and has just read the word "Zoloft" on the pill as if it's the lead story in *USA Today*. Then he immediately mouths the word "Zoloft" to everyone else at the table and pretty soon everyone you know thinks you're depressed or a basket case. Then you have to send out a mass e-mail explaining that you're not depressed, just a piñata filled with angst and panic and an assortment of other things that aren't good for you and that these pills just might help you relax and have better relations with people and they shouldn't judge you and you'd like to peek inside *their* medicine cabinets and you bet even if they're not taking any meds they at least have NyQuil!

My palms started itching even more than pre-Tamm. And the itching was inching up my forearms, approaching my elbow. I grabbed a container of fresh-squeezed orange juice, popped that little blue pill in my mouth and it slid down my throat like a prepubescent on a waterslide. Then I took a nap.

Miraculously, after a couple of weeks, I began to notice significant changes. For the first time in my life, the world seemed calm and pleasant and I had no urge to rush. I felt truly at peace, as if I had died and was staring at myself from above with a fresh perspective, finally behaving as I should. I looked forward to the minutiae of the wedding plans with Nancy, insisting on helping in every phase—even the flowers, though I still believe blue asters are a big waste of money. Road rage wasn't a passenger when I was driving. Unreturned business calls were shrugged off. Other people didn't bother me as much, if at all. I was actually slowing down my life and savoring it. I was finally healthy—three-dimensionally, not just on paper. That delightful drug sent messages throughout my body that gave me the revelation that perhaps *I* was the problem in my interpersonal relationships—not necessarily every other human I interacted with, as I had long suspected. *I* was the bull in a china shop. *I* was out of control. When Nancy noticed a Zoloftesque difference in my behavior, I attributed it to deep breathing, not something smaller than a Skittle that I kept in a bottle hidden in the back of my sock drawer.

I wanted to put all my money into Pfizer, the maker of Zoloft. I believe had Ron Artest been on Zoloft, he never would have gone into the stands in Detroit and punched those people; I believe had Milosevic been on Zoloft, there would have been no Bosnian conflict; I believe had Jeffrey Dahmer been on Zoloft, his freezer would have been stuffed with Omaha steaks instead of people's heads.

I wish I could have told my secret to everyone on the planet. I'd have done an infomercial with Tony Little. I'd have broadcast the cure for hyper-chondria on satellite TV to uptight, ill people in foreign lands. I could be the poster boy for Zoloft! I would work for them for free in gratitude for their outstanding product. But I had promised Dr. Tamm that I would keep my mouth shut. And he was my new hero.

So things were going pretty great for me and my serotonin-modified brain. I got married, shook my non-itchy hands with people who gave us wedding checks and went on a lovely erectile dysfunction–free honeymoon.

About a month after our wedding, I decided to tell Nancy. I couldn't keep making up reasons for the new and improved me. Besides, it's better to lie to your dermatologist than your wife.

"Nance, I have something to tell you."

"You've cheated already?"

"No. My dermatologist gave me some . . ."

"Retin-A?"

"No. Zoloft. I've been on it since March."

"Oh. I had no idea skin doctors could give out non-skin stuff."

"They can."

"Good for you!"

She was verging on jubilant about my newfound chemical reliance. My new spouse already had a commanding lead on me in calm and wouldn't have minded if I caught up a little. "Let

me know if I can do anything," her Joyce DeWitt face and petite nonconfrontational frame offered. "I can even pick up your
pills when I'm getting my Starbucks."

For eight-twelfths of a year, life in Los Angeles was good.
Nancy and I had both left *Blind Date* and discovered the joys of
writing sentences that didn't fit inside thought-bubbles. I
broke into magazines and she got her dream job of writing on a
sitcom, which came with my dream—better health insurance.
Though, ironically, I wasn't getting sick anymore. The only
side effect I had from Zoloft was calm.

Then one autumn afternoon, life got a lot less good.

I was driving along some curvy hillside roads when a guy in a
Honda Accord coming from the opposite direction drifted into
my lane, nearly forcing my car into a telephone pole. He then
stopped his car and fervently displayed his middle finger to the
apparent delight of the sneering collie in his passenger seat. I
should have just returned the gesture and kept driving, but I
couldn't. Instantly, it felt as if my Zoloft had lost its power. I was
on my own again, in charge of navigating my sea of rage.

I pulled a U-turn and tailgated Honda-man, determined to
make sure he was never again able to make one of his fingers
very tall. I stayed inches behind his car until it stopped at a
dog park, then I got out and chased that fucker across a soccer
field while simultaneously telling him I wanted to rip his head
off his neck. I was quite the multitasker. With my face two
inches away from his face, I could feel the words from my
threats bounce off his skin and ricochet back at me as the veins
in my neck and forehead popped out like a series of cuckoo
clocks. I was bordering on an aneurysm. The scary thing is, it
probably wouldn't have mattered who was driving that car
with the collie; it could've been Mike Tyson and my reaction
would have been the same. Because I hadn't been in a fight
since high school (which I lost), I spared the quivering collie
owner and his devoted pet. Then I went home and collapsed in
bed for the next fourteen hours. Meltdowns are exhausting.

The next morning, my neck hurt, my jaw throbbed and I felt as if I had an ulcer: the first signs of body malfunction since my hands stopped itching. My hyper-chondria was back.

I returned to my Zoloft dealer and Dr. Tamm immediately doubled my prescription. I would now be assigned to the light yellow 100 mg pill. (Which made it much harder for dining companions to read the word "Zoloft.") But the downside: the maximum recommended dose is 200 mg per day, so after a little less than a year, I was already halfway there. I did some quick math and realized that in another couple of years, I'd be immune to this entire selective serotonin reuptake inhibitor family—unless they developed a pill the size of my head. Then what the hell would I do? Switch to another stopgap drug like Paxil or Lexapro? Have kava root injected into my medulla? Maybe my podiatrist would prescribe electroshock therapy?

On my way to the pharmacy to pick up my new and improved prescription, a guy cut me off without signaling and I flipped out again and tailgated him through five traffic lights. Is this how insane I had been for the first thirty-nine years of my life? If so, it was a miracle I was a fully functioning adult with dozens of friends, girlfriends and now a wife. I needed a Zoloft IV on the way to get my Zoloft.

After being bumped up to the 100 mg pills I quickly noticed I wasn't twice as calm as when I was on the 50 mg pills; nor was I a hundred times as calm as in my pre-Zoloft days. Because my body had gotten used to the drugs, the double dose was now merely the equivalent of the single dose—way back when I first started taking it almost a year ago. Although my days on this stuff were numbered, it bought me time to look elsewhere for a more permanent, drug-free solution. The only trouble was, not a lot of time.

Since I finally knew what feeling peaceful and relaxed actually was like—and that it could be achieved within the confines of my body—I wanted to get back to that state. I was going to get to the bottom of this. I had to hurry up and calm down.

PART ONE

0 mg

1

YELLING

"Jesus Christ!"

"Jesus Christ yourself!!!!"

My parents yelled "Jesus Christ" at each other a minimum of fifteen times a day despite the fact that we were Jews.

It hadn't always been like this. Before my mother was diagnosed with multiple sclerosis my parents didn't fight much. But when I turned ten the house became a war zone. The screaming coupled with the constant barrage of doors slamming might as well have been gunshots.

"Sam! This isn't the jacket I wanted! I asked you to get me the *red* one! You do NOT listen!"

The disease had transformed my mother ostensibly overnight from an independent, warm, thoughtful first-grade teacher to an angry, frustrated woman who couldn't get her shoes on without assistance. Before MS invaded our household, I'm not sure there was a better mom on the planet. My mother, who looks like a Sheepshead Bay version of Audrey Hepburn, was beloved by her students and worshipped by our family. She wrote and directed new plays combining pop culture and fairy tales for her first-graders every year. She would read to my younger sister and me each night in a smooth, melodic voice reminiscent of radio commercials one would hear in the 1950s. She'd take us to arts and crafts shops weekly so we could do little projects (such as making hippopotamuses out of mini pompoms) and drive us to Marsh's or Macy's and let us pick out clothes for school that were far more expensive than what we could afford. But the MS took all of that away, and more.

Since she felt helpless and relied heavily on my father for

simple tasks like getting out of bed and using the bathroom, her pride took a hit. Even as a child, I could sense the embarrassment she felt at losing her independence as I was gaining mine. To compensate, my mother managed to package the endearing troika of being very demanding, very impatient and very irritated. And not only did she yell a lot, but objects were flung around as if we lived in an arthritic Foley studio. She had just turned thirty-seven.

For some reason, I always seemed to be in the thick of things. My brother, Mark, had the room adjacent to my parents, but because he was seventeen he wasn't around much. He had just become an Eagle Scout and happily spent much of his time sleeping in the woods with his troop. My sisters shared a room downstairs, but the older of the two, Debbie, had just turned fifteen and discovered the glamour of dating boys with driver's licenses. She preferred to be driven around in a Trans Am by a guy with a mustache and Black Sabbath thumping from a half-dozen speakers than to be exposed to the unmelodic shrieking of angry Jews. Meanwhile, my younger sister, Stacey, six, could be found huddled in the corner of the top bunk bed rereading *The Phantom Tollbooth* with cotton balls stuffed into each ear.

My room was upstairs directly across the hall from the madness and because I didn't know anyone with a Trans Am yet, nor was I interested in learning how to tie fifteen different kinds of knots, I was always around. And, since frustration is easily transferable, I was especially susceptible. Every syllable of fury permeated my tiny skull and would be stored inside for later use.

As bad as I felt for my mom, I felt even worse for my dad. Although he always dropped whatever he was doing if my mother needed something, it never seemed to be fast enough—and as in a video game, one little mistake would wipe out everything positive that had been accomplished. If he brought her home a pastrami sandwich, picked up all her prescriptions and did her laundry but mistakenly handed her a Diet Fresca instead of a Tab, my mother would unleash her wrath: an onslaught of constant reminders of how unlucky she was, how much pain she was in and how she couldn't wait to die. I sometimes wished I would go first.

Despite this harsh treatment, whenever my father was out running errands he'd rush back to be at my mother's side in case she needed anything or an emergency arose. Or maybe he was just scared of the repercussions of returning "late."

The owner of curly blond hair, a Fred MacMurray face and Popeye-sized forearms, my dad grew up in the Great Depression. His parents had emigrated from Poland in the early 1920s to escape the pogroms and had filled him with fear. He was never allowed to learn how to ride a bike or swim (both too dangerous) and even now he's scared to death to drive over bridges or at night, and forget about bridges at night. He's also afraid to shower or bathe and thus rarely does either. Whether this is symptomatic of his fear of water or of the prisoners' fate at Treblinka, or he just likes to be dirty, no one's quite sure. At the age of seventy-three, he still hasn't eaten a slice of pizza because my grandparents were convinced that any pizza parlor in Brooklyn would funnel the profits back to Mussolini in Italy who would then subsequently transfer the funds to the Nazis to be used against the Jews. Apparently this elaborate plan even included garlic knots. To this day, my father screams regularly in his sleep from nightmares of Nazis chasing him.

Perhaps because of all his fears, my dad immersed himself in the world of Golden Age comic books. When he was a kid he would run down to the corner store and buy every comic he could get his hands on: Superman, Batman, Action Comics, Plastic Man, The Star-Spangled Kid, The Flash, Captain Marvel, Captain America. If there was a guy with a cape on the cover, the comic would find a way into his bedroom. However, for some mysterious reason his collection peaked and then began to dwindle. No matter how many comics he bought, they continued disappearing faster than he could replenish

them. Finally, he discovered the cause. Whenever my dad was
out playing stickball, my grandmother would throw a few out.
She had no idea he'd even notice; cleanliness was more important to her than the latest exploits of Clark Kent.

So whether to relive his childhood, feel protected or just
ward off evil, my father was the only adult in town who still
collected comic books and was obsessed with superheroes. He
wore a Justice League of America jacket—even when it was
way too hot for a jacket of any kind; a baseball hat with the
Mighty Thor proudly displaying a large hammer was a fixture
atop his head; and he always wore a large pewter Superman
ring on his right hand with a giant *S* on it, decades before Hollywood started sinking its teeth into the comic book genre.

"Sam! Get up here! You forgot your Superman ring!" my
mother would shout. (In later years they rigged up an intercom
system so my father would transform into Pavlov's dog whenever he heard a buzzing sound.)

"Just a second, Rhoda!"

Then he'd charge up the fifteen stairs and enter the bedroom, crawling on the ground in slow motion.

"Too weak . . . need . . . ring . . . have . . . lost . . . all . . . superpowers!"

"You're an idiot, Sam!"

My mother didn't laugh a lot, at least in her current condition. So being called an idiot was the equivalent of a round of
applause at a comedy club.

She probably could've used a drink, but that wasn't an option in our house. My parents have had a total of four drinks
over the last three decades (two Old Milwaukees, a White
Russian and a frozen piña colada). And cursing was nearly as
rare. We probably had the highest yelling/squeaky-clean language ratio of any household in America. Four-letter words
were prohibited under any circumstances. Approximately once
a year, somebody would go absolutely nuts and spell "shit"
aloud. "Your father is such an S-H-I-T!" my mother would say,
in a cadence barely above a whisper.

Luckily, I didn't have to worry about too many of my friends being exposed to the tension emanating from each room, because it was rare that I had anyone over. I blamed it on Rufus, our Old English sheepdog, named after an innocuous character on *Sesame Street*. As a puppy in his pre-Frazer days, Rufus was cuddly and friendly, but he quickly transformed into a bona fide attack dog from living with our family. And one day he snapped. A cable TV man went into our backyard when we weren't home, ignoring both the leaping, overtly aggressive, loud-barking ninety-five-pound shaggy dog baring pointy teeth *and* the large-font Beware of Dog sign displayed prominently on the fence. Rufus tore him apart in about twenty seconds and my family had to go to court. Although we won the case, my mother blamed me for the incident, since I was the one who wanted cable.

In addition to my parents' behavior, I was aesthetically ashamed of my house. The common areas were all exceedingly messy and the carpets threadbare and stained. And, unlike any of my friends' homes, ours consisted solely of antiques. I made all my phone calls from an old 1943 rotary pay phone inside a 1927 phone booth with a glass accordion door that shut for optimum privacy. I watched television lying horizontally in a 1902 red vinyl–covered barber chair and checked the time on a 1936 neon bank clock that was the size of a small desk. There was a giant movie poster for *Down to Earth* starring Rita Hayworth from 1947 above a Woolworth's Five & Ten sign from 1931; velour movie theater seats from the 1940s sat next to a Ringling Brothers' drum from 1908. On the extraordinary occasion when we had any guests or relatives over, my dad would plug in the 1938 Wurlitzer jukebox, deposit a nickel from a nearby 1920s pickle jar and we'd hear the Andrews Sisters singing "Don't Sit Under the Apple Tree" or Peggy Lee crooning "Rum and Coca-Cola." I know, it may sound pretty cool now, but when you're growing up you just want some modern shit in your house like everybody else.

My mom's main joy in life had been reduced to buying antiques through mail-order catalogs, but she may have been even more gleeful when yelling at my father while he attempted to hang the nostalgia on the wall.

"It's not straight, Sam!"

"It is straight, Rhoda. I measured it."

I would always take my father's side. He'd gone to college on an art scholarship and began his career teaching it. He also made money on the side doing calligraphy and transforming wedding and bar mitzvah photographs into pen-and-ink drawings. When it came to hanging things he had the magic eye.

"Cool Yer Pitz, Ma!"

This was Debbie's method of restoring order, but her proclamation just got everybody more riled up.

"Don't you DARE tell me to cool my pitz!" my mother thundered. "You cool *your* pitz!"

"No, you cool *yours*!"

"Deb-bie! I am *not* speaking to you anymore!" And my mother and Debbie would ignore each other for the next month. The silent treatment was actually far more intense than any bellowing because you can't fight silence with more silence. So whoever had initiated the silence held all the power. It was, in fact, a brilliant tactical maneuver, albeit a destructive one.

"Sam, I am *tel-ling* you"—my mother would break even the simplest of words apart to emphasize her point—"it is not *straight*!"

"What part of it isn't straight?"

"The *who-le* thing."

And on and on the argument would go until he'd moved the piece around on the wall like a pointer on a Ouija board, eventually circling back to where it had originally been hung. Only now, my mother would take the credit for its perfectly symmetrical position.

"Now it is *strai-ght*, Sam!"

Besides arguing with my father about minutiae, my mother's main source of solace was shopping. However, she rarely left the house and going to a store to try on clothes was out of the question. Practically every other day the UPS man would be at our door requesting a signature, and every other day my dad would be at the mall returning or exchanging merchandise my mother had charged through catalogs. Her purchases were based solely on a two-inch photo on glossy paper, so inevitably, 90 percent of them wound up being the wrong size, a poor fit, of inferior quality or exactly as the catalog advertised but she had changed her mind. As my mother's condition worsened, her catalog shopping increased dramatically and my father's trips to the mall exponentially. Our "family" trips to the plethora of indoor stores weren't exactly relaxing either. But when you're ten or eleven years old and you still don't drive, you're at the mercy of whoever has car keys.

When David Sywak's parents drove us to the mall, they'd give us a minimum of an hour to look around and then meet them back at a designated spot. Mr. Hastings even gave us two hours. My dad: fifteen minutes. Fifteen minutes? In a friggin' mall?!?! You've gotta be kidding! But he wasn't. "But Mr. Frazer," my friends would plead, "there are over a hundred stores here!"

"Yes," replied my father, in his deep monotone schoolteacher voice. "But some of them sell things that won't interest you."

Since we had little choice but to obey the rules, my friends and I had to run around like prepubescent madmen to Spencer Gifts and that store that just sold purple things, and no matter how much we rushed, we always seemed to be at least a minute late, which irritated my dad. And forget about trying to buy anything. Unless there was a combination of no line *and* a cashier who was actually lucid and competent, no matter how fast we ran around, there was little chance of having any transaction take place and getting to our red VW bug on time.

With all his rushing and stress, why didn't my father have hyper-chondria? Maybe because he *couldn't* get sick. If he did, we'd all die. Or at least starve, since he did all the food shopping.

Being hyper, I learned, seemed a surefire way to please my mother. It was certainly the method that would result in the least criticism and anger. Her chief complaint was that nothing she needed was ever done fast enough. And when you're lying in bed all day, it's tough to argue with that. Ironically, it would seem that since she didn't need to rush around and actually *be* anywhere at any given time, slow would be just as preferable. But it wasn't. Time became a different entity that was measured not in minutes and seconds but in units of pain and discomfort. Her theory (which was soon to be mine) was that there was no use in putting things off because you'd eventually have to do them anyway. So, at the tender age of eleven, I became ultra task-oriented. I made lists of things I needed to accomplish, and if a writing utensil wasn't handy to cross items out, I'd tear off the part of the paper that contained the task I had just completed, eventually rendering the mighty eight-by-ten-inch sheet into a fortune-cookie-sized sliver. I walked Rufus after he had barely started eating; if I was asked to vacuum the living room and load the dishwasher, each chore was done before anyone had even thought it was started; when assigned a book report in school, I'd read the entire thing that night (although by the time we'd discuss it in class, I'd have forgotten pretty much everything but the title); if it snowed I was outside shoveling as the first flake hit. As far as I was concerned, my mother's logic was flawless.

2

FOAMING

I wasn't too keen about Hebrew school. It seemed like a stupid, boring waste of time. Besides, with blond hair and blue eyes, everyone assumed I was Irish anyway. The kids at school referred to me as "Hitler's Favorite Jew," which for a group of eleven-year-olds was actually quite creative.

Even as a prepubescent, the mere thought of organized religion spooked me. I actually flinched if someone even said the word "pray." I didn't believe that begging God for things did any good; otherwise, my grandparents wouldn't have been beaten up in the Polish pogroms of World War I, my aunts and uncles wouldn't have been killed in Treblinka, my father wouldn't still be having Nazi nightmares and my thirty-seven-year-old mother would've been able to walk to the bathroom without the aid of two aluminum canes. But I went because (a) I had no choice in the matter and (b) Janice Jacoby was going and she already needed a bra.

I wish I could say that I enjoyed myself for those three years, but I didn't. I hated everything about Hebrew school—the musty smells inside the temple, wearing that tiny brimless hat, the assortment of phlegmy sounds everyone was forced to make. But apparently, I'd be less of a man if I didn't stick with the program.

Then there was the other issue. Every syllable leaving my mouth was slurred, mumbled and garbled. I'd been going to an assortment of speech therapists since first grade, and despite my diligence, my impediment had barely improved over the ensuing seven years. I just kept practicing the same verbal exercises with no guidance or adjustments from any of my therapists. It wasn't until I was a freshman in college that my designated instructor got to the root of the problem: my tongue was too big for my mouth. I should have realized this without any outside assistance since I could easily pick my nose with my tongue—a handy party trick to pull out in college, but not the boon with the ladies you'd think. "Not only is your tongue too large," I was finally told, at age nineteen, by Dr. Sharon Reingold, "but when you speak, it's aimlessly flailing around in your mouth. Your tongue is unruly and hyperactive, dear." Once again, my troubles stemmed from trying to do things too fast.

To avoid mumbling in Hebrew in front of my peers and family, I neglected my lessons, so much so that my bar mitzvah was in danger of being postponed. In her shrinking, bedridden world, my mother had a lot of time for overanalyzing. A belated bar mitzvah would embarrass the family, particularly her, and she would have no choice but to unleash her ire upon the chief culprit—me. She alternated between power yelling and the silent treatment with the speed of a changing traffic light. I couldn't have been more frightened if she had pointed a knife at me.

These tactics would be immediately followed by her unjustly blaming the entire situation on my father, who would then mope around the house like a miniature schnauzer who'd been hit with a Sunday newspaper, causing guilt to trickle back down to me a second time. Simultaneously, my mother would manage to scream about "your fath-er and broth-er!" to my three siblings, who would in turn yell back at me because this time I was responsible for igniting the powder keg of rage. It was easier to just bite the bullet and become a man on time.

Fortunately, my rabbi cut me a deal.

Rabbi Setzman was in his mid-thirties and proudly wore a large fluffy mustache above his lip. He resembled a Semitic Tony Orlando with a paler entourage.

"Brian, you need to put more time into this or you won't have your special day."

"Oh."

"But I'm willing to stay late and meet you here a few nights a week so you can learn your haftorah. All you have to do is promise to continue coming to temple for another year after your bar mitzvah."

That didn't sound like a very good deal. The rabbi would give up a couple of his boring rabbi nights and I'd have to sacrifice another year of my effervescent adolescence. But I couldn't afford to haggle with the mustachioed Jew. We shook hands as if we were at a Camp David summit and the deal was done.

After several weeks of one-on-one tutoring—which required transporting truckloads of saliva from the back of my throat to the front of my mouth in a language I didn't speak nor would ever use outside the temple walls—I pulled it together and my big day was back on schedule.

"You really came through." The rabbi smiled. "I'm proud of you."

"Thanks," I mumbled.

Then he reached into the inside pocket of his tweed sports jacket and handed me a small box.

"This is for all your hard work."

At first I thought I had committed a faux pas by not getting the rabbi anything, as if we had drawn each other in Secret Santa.

I opened the box hoping there was a Tom Seaver baseball card inside, which was unlikely since Tom Terrific wasn't one of the Chosen People. But I'd certainly settle for a Kenny Holtzman rookie card. On either account, I was far off the mark.

"Wow!" I said with mock appreciation. "A Star of David! On a chain!"

"It's pewter. Go ahead, try it on. One size fits all." The rabbi chuckled.

I wasn't much into jewelry. This was at least a decade before even the coolest of kids had earrings and I had never been one to wear a bracelet, or even a watch. But there was something about this star that was special. I put it around my neck and felt proud. It was a symbol of all my hard Jew-man-like work and I had no plans of ever taking it off. I was now officially in the same club as Hank Greenberg, Dolph Schayes, and several other obscure athletes in the *Great Jewish Sports Heroes* book (actually more like a pamphlet) that I had purchased in the synagogue gift shop.

I walked around our house with my chest arched forward like a peacock, so nobody could possibly miss my new accoutrement of splendor.

"Hey, whatcha got there?" Mark asked.

I was always cognizant of keeping my answers to my brother terse, so he would have fewer of my unintelligible words to mock. It seemed that anything I said was easy prey for Mark's perfectly pitched, deep radio voice—which he would later use on-air in his career as an oldies DJ.

"Rabbi gift." I figured two words would limit his ammunition.

"Cool beans!"

I never understood exactly what this meant, but he said it a lot and it was apparently a good thing.

After being home for all of ten minutes, I began doing something that would haunt me for the better part of 1977; I began grinding that six-pointed star of pewter directly into my sternum. Over and over and over again. Really really hard. And I couldn't stop. When I tired of grinding one of the points, I had five others at my disposal. I would then rotate the star counterclockwise and continue my cleavage rampage.

Nervous habits were nothing new for me—I'd always had one. I bit my nails for three years. I twirled my hair for a summer. But neither of those habits seemed very original. Or heterosexual. Besides, there was something oddly soothing about all the star-induced discomfort. Perhaps it was a feeble attempt to compete for my mother's monopoly on pain. Or, as others now tell me, a cry for attention. Bottom line, it felt damn good.

My bar mitzvah day arrived and I fumbled through numerous sections of the Torah, occasionally forgetting to read things right to left, but I suspect only the rabbi and a distant relative from Tel Aviv knew of my incompetence. Off the pulpit, I was even less smooth. Because I hadn't been schooled in bar mitz-vah etiquette, I soon learned that one is *not* supposed to open up the card and pocket the cash the moment a guest hands you an envelope. However, despite my collection of temple gaffes, I could now open a savings account. Janice Jacoby had commem-orated the event by wearing a tight red frilly shirt. It was defi-nitely all "cool beans."

A week later, my father got a telephone call—which was un-usual in itself. Even though he's one of the nicest, kindest, friendliest humans ever, my father had no friends. Zero. His life was way too chaotic to leave time for anyone outside the family. I had heard about his best friend from childhood, Chop-sie, who now lived in St. Louis, but I had never met the guy. I don't even remember Chopsie ever calling the house, nor can I recall my father ever calling him. Perhaps it was better to have no friends than one friend named Chopsie. Once in a while my father would get a call from a stranger who had received his self-published comic book catalog in the mail and wanted to see if Spider-Man number 11 or Fantastic Four number 36 was still available to purchase, but that was the extent of his phone life. And I'm sure of this because it was really easy to monitor his phone calls.

When my mother, brother or sisters got a call and someone else answered, the *second* they picked up the phone they'd yell the standard "I got it!!!!" and then wouldn't utter another word until they heard the person who answered hang up. But my father either didn't understand the concept of eavesdrop-ping or didn't care if anyone else listened. If he got a call and I had nothing better to do, I would listen from another phone to the entire conversation (which, like I said, was always about whether Hawkman number 41 was *really* in mint condition or the specifics of Little Lulu number 23's spine damage). But I had a feeling this call was something even more important than superheroes because my father's phone voice was always monotone and for once he was actually transmitting a cadence.

All I heard him say was: "Hello? What? Jesus Christ!"

It was Marlene Oppenheimer from temple with some news. Rabbi Setzman had quit the synagogue because he was becoming an Episcopalian minister and moving to Woonsocket, Rhode Island, on Friday. The entire community was shocked. Rabbis don't usually resign, especially those in their mid-thirties in good health. Only a month ago this guy had bar mitzvahed me! Torah this, torah that, Jews Jews Jews . . . blah blah blah. And now the ultimate betrayal. And what about our agreement? I had to promise to go to temple for an extra year, but Mr. Rabbi could just bolt whenever he pleased?!

What was it that made Setzman suddenly change his mind and switch religions? I mean, if he was having doubts about his faith, the least he could've done is quit the temple and mull things over for a while. He performed my bar mitzvah on a Saturday, quit the temple on a Monday, and by Tuesday renounced Judaism, dropped off his yarmulke collection at Goodwill and picked up a box of communion wafers to munch on the drive up to Woonsocket. That meant that he probably started to have a change of heart a few months *before* he actually converted—I mean nobody can just flip-flop that quickly. So while I was being bar mitzvahed, my rabbi was probably up on the pulpit thinking about Jesus! Not cool. No wonder God had punished my mother; we were being rabbied by a fraud!!! I removed the Star of David from my neck immediately.

But that didn't stop me from grinding something else into my chest. The index finger on my right hand immediately enlisted and kept up the onslaught against my sternum. And the dent kept getting deeper. Nothing could make me stop the violence against myself. It was as if I had sprinkled a healthy smattering of birdseed on my chest and then invited a woodpecker over for dinner.

Believe me, it's tough enough hitting puberty and getting horny for the first time *without* compulsively tapping the center of your torso every waking hour. I was a freak. Katie Berkal thought so, as did Marcie Kaplan. "Why do you keep touching your chest?" they asked. "Uh . . ." I stammered, "because I can't touch yours?" The real reason: I was a nervous wreck. And not the kind that lies at the bottom of the sea and quivers, like the joke on the Dixie cup.

My parents became concerned and sent me to the family physician, which I was pretty psyched about. Dr. Torino always seemed to have the right answers for my ailments. When I continued going to school week after week with a small Band-Aid covering wherever the largest pimple on my face happened to be, he prescribed extra-strength acne medication; when I contracted pityriasis rosea, a rare skin disease, he gave me some free erythromycin and Cortaid; and years later, when I was in college living in an ancient dorm that banned refrigerators because of the fragile electrical system, he wrote me a note claiming that I required fresh, cold citrus juices and I became the only student in the building with a legal Kenmore.

When Dr. Torino saw the small hole I was creating in my chest, he arrived at a simple solution: he taped a gauze pad over my sternum to cushion the blows. As he handed my father a large stack of replacement pads, he turned to me: "This should hold you for a while. In the meantime, go back to biting your nails or something."

"I'll try," I said as I discreetly sneaked my hand up my shirt to peck myself.

For the next week I walked around school with a gauze pad under my shirt. But little else had changed. I continued to grind my index finger smack into the center of my chest. Only now, the gauze pad made things worse. I took it as a challenge to break through the cottony square, as if it were the last level of Arkanoid. When it was evident that a single pad wasn't doing the trick, Dr. Torino suggested that we up the ante and add another.

Before long I was walking around school with four or five gauze pads stacked on top of each other and taped to my sternum under my Huckapoo shirts. People started to ask me what was wrong. "Nothing," I said. "Just a little infection." Marcie Kaplan pointed, stared and giggled. I told Katie Berkal that the pads on my chest were from the nurse, to dispense in case anyone hurt themselves. That was the last time Katie Berkal ever spoke to me.

By the time seventh grade turned into eighth, the dent in my sternum had turned into a crater. My parents decided that my grinding problem needed to grind to a halt. And that is how I met Dr. Robert Spikol of Mineola, New York. Hypnotist. The first in a long line of charlatans proffering alternative treatments. For a mere $75 a session he would allow me to touch my sternum while I became sleepy.

I sat in a small dark room in the world's most comfortable chair. It was upholstered in soft brown leather—probably made from the planet's three laziest cows—and it reclined and had speakers on the headrest and you just sank right into it like quicksand. I swear to God I would have fucked that thing if Dr. Spikol wasn't in the room. Or if I knew how to fuck.

Dr. Spikol had dark red wavy hair, a closely cropped beard and small round glasses that made him look very clever. His gravelly voice emerged from both speakers as I sat there for an hour, drifting in and out of sleep. I thought it was all a waste of time but figured I needed to try anything to preserve my chest cavity. Plus, this gave my father a chance to do some pen-and-ink drawings of empty chairs in the waiting room.

After our first session, Dr. Spikol shook his head. He had been a hypnotist for twenty-eight years and called me the most hyper, high-strung patient he had ever had—which, thanks to Dr. Tamm, I now know to be a bad thing. But back in eighth grade I thought I had just won a contest and would receive a small trophy.

"You have to learn how to relax or your life is going to be a very short one."

I didn't realize that the $75 an hour included threats.

"I'm trying to." Actually, I really wasn't. At that point in my life, calm versus not calm was a completely foreign concept. Plus, the fact that I had recently weaned myself off the Beatles and discovered the joy of punk didn't help any. To me, the late '70s were the glory years of music—the Ramones, Talking Heads, the Clash. The riffs were powerful, explosive and full of energy—in hindsight all of which I could have probably done without. It was impossible to have your alarm clock go off in the morning with a Buzzcocks song playing on WLIR and not maniacally spring out of bed.

After several sessions of hearing Dr. Spikol's bleating voice transmitted through the chair, I was given a pair of light yellow foam blocks, each about the size of a cigarette lighter.

"These blocks are essential to your well-being."

"Uh . . . what am I supposed to do with them?" I had thought maybe they were magical insoles to insert in my shoes.

"Carry them around with you at all times."

"At all times?"

"Yes."

"In my pockets?"

"No. In your hands. You are NOT to put these blocks down unless eating, sleeping or showering."

"Wow."

"You need to keep your hands busy in a nondestructive manner at all times."

"Okay. I'll do it."

So now I had evolved from the freak with the jackhammer attached to his wrist to the freak palming foam.

I carried those things around school scrunched up in my hands so tightly that I suspect nobody knew I had tiny rectangular palm-sized blocks stashed in there. However, they probably *did* think that I was perpetually angry (which I was), since each of my hands was always arranged in a fist. Which again probably didn't help any with the ladies. It was nearly impossible to be cool around Laura Gesner with both hands empty, let alone clasping foam.

Unfortunately, the forearm bash had not been invented yet, so it was also difficult to greet my friends. Instead, I accomplished this with a mere jerk of my head, as if I were a giant Pez dispenser. Occasionally I would shake hands with someone in the hallway, which required extra dexterity. I had to slyly remove the foam from one hand and slide it into a back pocket, kind of like that one-armed pitcher Jim Abbott when he shoved his mitt under his stub to make a throw.

Once, while I was attempting this maneuver with Lyle Hastings, one of the blocks fell out of my hands and I was forced to explain what they were for.

"My hypnotist gave them to me to keep my hands off my chest."

Lyle thought it was cool and wanted to sign my foam, as if it were a cast. I turned him down. I didn't need any additional foreign substances on it. Because no matter how often I washed my hands, the blocks continued to get filthier and filthier. I replaced them several times by going to an art supply store and having my father cut chunks of foam into hand-sized pieces, but the mounting grime seemed to accelerate. Not only were they turning black, but I couldn't keep miscellaneous pen ink from infiltrating them, which frequently caused trouble. During tests, teachers would see these ink-stained, mucky, off-yellow pieces of foam on my desk and believe I was using them to cheat. Once they were even confiscated, but swiftly returned when Mr. Lennett determined that none of the random marks of filth had anything to do with Medieval History.

For the most part, I kept the foam in my hands as I was told, and as dumb as it sounds, it worked. Whenever I held the blocks, I felt calm and at peace with the world. And they kept my sternum safe from myself. At least through the summer before ninth grade when I cut my ring finger on a Shasta can and ink and filth seeped into the cut and my hand got infected and I had no choice but to throw away the foam for good.

Luckily I would soon have something else to occupy my hands.

3

GAMBLING

Foam or no foam, women aren't exactly drawn to hyperchondriacs. And my mumbling didn't help.

I became so self-conscious that in tenth grade I stopped talking to girls in my high school and relegated my search for dates to young ladies from surrounding areas who wouldn't know of my grinding, garbled past. Fortunately, I played in a basketball league with some kids from nearby schools, one of whom had a sister who sometimes came to our games. One night, after not having a sucky fourth quarter, I asked her out. She said yes. Finally, at the age of sixteen I had struck gold! I was in shock. Not only that a girl would say yes but that she actually understood the question I had asked.

Lisa Kulaska became the first girl I would pick up in my cream-colored Firebird, which I'd just hand-waxed. She was tall, lanky and had indecisive hair that didn't seem to know in what style it would settle, and I was desperate to impress her— which is hard to do when you work part-time at the Rusty Scupper washing dishes for $4 an hour.

I didn't want to take her to the typical Long Island teen date place like Friendly's. Everyone did that. It would have to be more extravagant. I arranged for a Friday night at Pizza City East and then the movie *Arthur* at the Manetto Hill Theater. One problem: it was already Tuesday and since all my dishwashing money went straight back into my car upkeep, insurance and gas, I didn't even have enough cash for a slice. I had four days to figure something out. As usual I needed to work fast.

o o o

The Hendersons looked smart. Especially Old Mr. Henderson. There was no way on earth that the Dohertys knew more. I was positive about that.

"I'll take the Hendersons for ten bucks."

"Sure."

I'd been introduced to betting the previous year during Super Bowl XIII when I put $5 on the Steelers against the Cowboys and won. It was empowering, making me feel like the ultimate multitasker. I could be at the Scupper washing dishes while Franco Harris's touchdown romp magically doubled my hourly wage. But this wasn't football season, so I had to get creative.

I invited myself over to Kenny Feldman's house on Tuesday and had just bet him money I didn't have that the Hendersons would be the winning family on that night's episode of *Family Feud*. The look in Mrs. Henderson's eyes told me I had done the right thing.

"Something that you pack in a suitcase?" bleated Richard Dawson.

"Uh . . . an iron . . ." said Grandpa Henry Henderson, who in hindsight looked like someone who didn't do very much traveling.

"A coffee mug . . ." Henry's daughter, the matronly Donna Henderson, insisted.

"No! No!" interrupted Donna's husband, Morton Henderson. "A throw rug!"

The Hendersons were idiots and now nearly three hours of future dishwashing dollars were down the drain. And, if this kept up, so might my dream Friday night with Lisa Kulaska. After *Family Feud* ended, Kenny and I switched over to *The Price Is Right*, but the results were the same. I lost. Which wouldn't have been so bad had I refrained from going double-or-nothing each time. I took a thrashing in "Plinko." Got dominated in "The Yodeler." Wiped out in "Higher or Lower." Then my debts doubled again on the "Showcase Showdown." I'd just assumed that the older people would win, since they had more experience buying things. Within an hour, I owed Kenny $160.

With only two more days before my date with Lisa, I now had
to pay off my debts to Kenny *and* come up with enough cash
for my big night. To compensate for my game-show-betting
deficiencies, I was about to pit my father's fantasy world against
mine.

As you may remember, my dad had an ever-expanding
comic book collection, not to mention a small mail-order catalog of thousands of titles for sale. Some were very valuable.
Kenny Feldman just so happened to like comic books. On
Wednesday afternoon, I invited "The Feld" over to my house
while my dad was at work so I could settle my debt. I let him
pick out some comics, like Captain Marvel number 17 or Batman number 21 . . . $160 worth of whatever he wanted that I
thought the man who raised me wouldn't miss. I even gave
Kenny extra comics to get some cash back for my date. I know.
I was an asshole. Thank God I wasn't married at sixteen or I
would've pawned Nancy's wedding ring.

With Batman money in hand and guilt in my head, I picked
up Lisa Kulaska and split a large pizza with four toppings and
some tiramisu. Then we were off to watch Dudley Moore act
like a drunk for ninety-one minutes. Halfway through the film,
I mustered up enough courage to fake-yawn and put my arm
around Lisa. And then I felt it, protruding from her body like
scaffolding.

"Whoaattaoosa?!"

"It's okay," she whispered reassuringly. "It's just my back
brace."

What? My first prospective girlfriend and she had a sharp
piece of metal the length of her spine strapped to her back with
large stiff pieces of canvas wrapped around her chest? No wonder she'd said yes when I asked her out. She was a physiological
misfit. Like me!

"Uh . . . can you take it off?" Everything I did was inept.

"No."

"Um . . . uh . . ." I shouldn't have been worried about the

words I chose. The chance of her understanding anything I mumbled was only 30 percent.

"What's . . . uh . . . wrong with it?"

"I have scoliosis. But the doctor says if I wear it for the next two years, my spine should straighten out so I won't have to bring it to college."

"Um . . . you wear it to class?"

"No. I have to wear it sixteen hours a day so I put it on as soon as I get home from school."

"So you wear it to bed?" I couldn't stop asking questions.

"Yeah, but I'm used to it."

I wasn't. How could I have missed the brace? It was as if she were a scarecrow hanging on a metal pole with that thing up the back of her shirt. What a hassle. But I couldn't break up with someone who was handicapped. That would be jerky of me. Then I felt guilty that there wasn't a mechanism that could be attached to my mother to make her walk again. Or at least something she could wear on her legs at night that would slowly rejuvenate them.

One thing for certain, it took all the pressure off what base Lisa and I would get to. I knew I couldn't get much farther than first. I didn't have a tool kit with me. God only knows how she managed to detach that thing from her torso. She probably had to involve her entire family, as if they were an Indy pit crew. As I clumsily leaned in for a kiss, my hands groped her back and my palms moved up and down the aluminum rod steering her spine. At one point I even thought I got a shard of metal in my thumb and would need a tetanus shot, which momentarily freaked me out.

Even though Lisa was a lousy kisser, I would definitely ask her out again. And take her somewhere even nicer, to prove her brace didn't bother me. I'd just have to come up with more money.

I was smart enough to realize that Kenny Feldman was out of my league. Luckily Louis Bevalaqua lived around the corner. Louis, a thirteen-year-old with a paper route, was my friend

Evan's chubby younger brother. I felt guilty that I was intro-
ducing a seventh-grader to gambling, but not guilty enough
not to do it. Besides, betting $50 a game on *$10,000 Pyramid*
would make him feel like a grown-up.

After an hour of Dick Clark correcting contestants' answers
and me losing more money, Mrs. Bevalaqua wanted to watch
her soap operas on the family's lone television. So the Bevalaqua runt and I headed off to his basement to see what else
we could gamble on. We decided on Yahtzee. And within seconds I became his Yahtzee bitch. No matter what I rolled, it
was either a duplicate of something I already had on my score
sheet or a useless set of dice that could only go into my
"Chance" column. Meanwhile, Louis was rolling not only
Yahtzees but four-of-a-kinds and straights. At one point I was
so discouraged, I actually put one of the dice to my ear and
shook it to make sure there wasn't some kind of trained insect
inside that Louis had taught to land on six.

But Louis hadn't rigged anything. He was just a damn good
Yahtzee player. After three days, I owed him nearly $850, $832
of which I didn't have—thanks to Kenny Feldman and the
non-lucrative world of getting plates clean. There was only one
thing to do . . .

Louis and I went into my basement and I let him pick out a
few hundred dollars' worth of comics. A Silver Surfer . . . an
original Human Torch . . . an old Hawkman. To decrease the
likelihood of my father noticing his stock had diminished from
"The Feld"'s take, I had packed the tomato cartons where he
stored his books with a variety of old mail-order catalogs from
Sears and Abraham & Strauss. And if he noticed anything missing, I could always blame it on his shoddy bookkeeping skills.
(Or on my grandmother, since she already had a record.) And
naturally, I gave Louis an extra Silver Surfer in exchange for
some cash. Now I was relying on a thirteen-year-old to fund
my dates.

Had Lisa learned that comic-pilfering was sponsoring the
mozzarella sticks, fried onion rings and virgin frozen piña co-

ladas she was enjoying on our second date, she probably would
have reported me to the police and never spoken to me again.
But as far as she was concerned, my dishwashing dollars fi-
nanced our fancy entertainment.

I should've just written my dad an IOU, quit gambling and
put my surplus energy into something more useful . . . like
homework. But I was like the prettiest girl at the dance.
Within days every kid in town wanted to bet with me. And
who could blame them? Not only did I lose most of the time,
but I always took my losses with grace, and on the rare occasions when I *did* win, I genuinely felt bad for the other guy.
Maybe deep down I didn't even care if I won; I just liked the
companionship, excitement and diversion from my home.

Lisa and I had date number three lined up for the following
Saturday night, which was why I couldn't say no to Eddie
Kunoff. Eddie and I were the perfect match for Mattel Electronic Football. He liked to take advantage of people with un-
coordinated thumbs and I liked to mortgage my future. So the
two of us played game after game after game for dollar after
dollar . . . few of which I won. Whether the batteries were fresh
or just about to die, I was no match for Eddie's nimble fingers.
They flicked mightily back and forth on that piece of plastic
that looked like a calculator, creating Hail Mary passes through
a maze of red dashes and specks. I swear his thumbs were on
steroids or something.

Over the course of four days, I lost fifty-five out of fifty-
eight games to Eddie. I think the three games I won were only
because he was distracted thinking about what he was going to
buy with all the money I owed him. Which was now in the
neighborhood of $1,700. It was actually in an even more ex-
pensive neighborhood, but Eddie said he'd take money off if I
helped him with his chores, which included moving some
heavy furniture for his mom. Carrying a credenza down thirteen stairs is way harder than it sounds.

When I got home post–credenza carrying, my left testicle

was burning and aching. At first I thought I might have a hernia. I didn't know what to do. My father wasn't home and even if he were, we'd always avoided anything even remotely related to sex. Once he and I were watching TV and a beer ad came on in which sexy women in bikinis played volleyball and drank beer. It was the most awkward thirty seconds I'd ever spent with anyone. At the end of the commercial, my dad turned to me and quivered, "I didn't know you were allowed to bring beer to the beach." So I would have to describe my latest malady to my mother, which, oddly enough, wasn't as embarrassing as I thought it would be.

"Um . . . I think there's something wrong with my . . . testicle."

"What?!"

"It's all lumpy and veiny and burns on one side."

"Sam!"

I was back at Dr. Torino's office. As he examined my ball, I wondered if he'd prescribe putting a gauze pad over it, as he did my sternum. After pressing his ear to my lower abdominal wall and tapping on it with his hands, he ruled out a hernia. Then he squeezed each of my balls simultaneously, as if he were picking out peaches or mini-tangerines. He looked up at me and informed me that I had a varicocele. I was told to take a lot of warm baths, not lift anything heavy for a few weeks and lie down if it flared up. And, since a varicocele can prevent sperm from passing through, I'd need to have my semen analyzed to make sure I was still fertile. I'm sixteen, for Chrissakes!!! Infertility? From being bad at Mattel Electronic Football and moving a friend's mom's dresser? Fuck! None of this would've happened had I just taken Lisa for a Fribble™ and not tried to be a big shot. So in a matter of weeks, I'd become a compulsive gambler, a kleptomaniac *and* had a droopy, veiny ball! Plus I still owed Eddie Kunoff nearly fifteen hundred bucks.

Most teenagers would have just forgotten about their debts, especially since the amounts being bet were ludicrous. But I was an honorable person, at least among people who didn't live in my house. Besides, as a compulsive gambler, I always thought my next bet would go in my favor and I'd dig myself out of the hole I'd created and buy back my dad's comics and everything would return to normal. Just the opposite happened. My debts grew and my father's comics shrank.

Then a very insane thought came into my head. One game, winner-take-all. Double-or-nothing. If I won, I wouldn't owe Eddie a cent. But if Eddie won . . . well . . . he'd get my father's *entire* comic book collection. I already figured out I'd suck up some of the blame by telling my parents we got robbed and that I *might* have forgotten to lock the front door while Rufus was in the backyard.

Why was I willing to sacrifice my father's prized Submariner comic based on how in sync my thumbs were in relation to a neighbor's? What was wrong with me? I later realized that I might have been trying to get back at my dad for being the ultimate Submariner, submerging his emotions. The truth is, he had to. If he let even a fraction of them out, he probably would've gone mad. Unfortunately, this also made him emotionally unavailable to us. But I couldn't blame him for that. It was his only way of coping.

Eddie and I hunkered down in his paneled rec room and I received the kickoff. I maneuvered my blip around the converging blips and flicked my thumbs around that little beige board as if I were having an epileptic seizure. At last, melodic chirps emanating from the one-inch speaker signified that I had scored a touchdown! Success! Then Eddie scored a touchdown while simultaneously popping a blackhead on his chin and listing the prettiest girls in our school in order. Then I scored again. And back and forth we went. Touchdown. Touchdown. Touchdown.

The first one to make a mistake would inevitably be the loser. And I assumed it would be me. I considered pressing the buttons really hard to try to break the game and then insist I'd won by default, since the upkeep of the toy should be Eddie's responsibility. Then the incredible happened. Kunoff threw an interception! I don't know if he felt sorry for me and my varicocele and did it on purpose or if that little defensive blip just out-deeked him. But I didn't care. All I had to do now was score from a scant twenty-two yards out and I'd have this thing in the bag.

He handed me the game, which nearly slipped out of my sweaty, panic-coated hands. As my heart's thumps matched the pulse of the game's thumps, my quarterback scrambled around, nearly getting sacked. Then miraculously, as if all the defensive blips had simultaneously pulled hamstrings, I managed to zigzag around every one of them until I had secured a first down, then continued along the sidelines for bonus yardage. I kept flailing my thumbs on the tiny directional squares in the hopes of hearing that loud buzz from the tiny Mattel speakers, indicating that the game was over. This meant that once I was tackled, that was it. I still had another ten yards to go. The pressure was unbearable as beads of sweat dripped from my forehead down onto the playing field, obscuring some of the players. Had this been Mattel Electronic Baseball, the grounds crew would've had to bring the tarp out. I had never been so frightened in my life. One inadvertent maneuver and my father would be superhero-less! Or worse, I'd have to sign over the title of my car. Either way, I'd never be able to afford to date again. My thumbs relentlessly slammed the squares as fast as they could until I heard the celebratory tones that indicated a score. Touchdown! The game was over and I was debt-free from Eddie. In fact, debt-free from everyone. And most important, my dad's comics wouldn't migrate twice in his lifetime.

I was so relieved I removed the batteries from Eddie's Mattel Electronic Football game and stuffed them into my pocket, so I wouldn't be tempted to play some more. I left the Kunoffs' rec room and, on my jubilant walk home, flung those double-A's down the sewer. And, despite my monumental losses, I felt as if I had gotten off easy.

But I hadn't. To get out of lugging more heavy furniture around to work off my debt, Eddie was the only person I had told about my varicocele and he assured me he'd keep it a secret. Not only did he not keep it a secret but he seemed to go out of his way to tell people. The story spread like brush fire in school. As I walked down the hallways, girls would giggle, point at my groin and scatter. Guys would mock me, both behind my back and to my face. "Hey, Frazer . . . you wanna play basketBALL!!!"

Then, forty-five minutes before I was going to leave to pick up Lisa, I got a phone call.

"I really like you," said Lisa, "but I think we should break up."

I nearly yelled out: Is it because of my ball! My hideous left ball?! It's my ball, isn't it?!! Instead I went for the more conventional, "Why?"

"Because . . . uh . . . I have to concentrate on Spanish."

I pondered over whether it was because she'd heard about my sick testicle or discovered my gambling addiction and was worried that she'd come home one day to find all her Shaun Cassidy posters missing. Or maybe it was my mumbling. All I know is, it wasn't because of Spanish because she told me at Pizza City that she took French.

Within a week, the angst and stress of being teased about my ball and dumped overwhelmed my body. I became so weak and queasy I was sent home from school. It was a struggle just to drive the three miles. I had searing abdominal pain, coughing fits, a high fever, chills.

After some small talk about my testicle, Dr. Torino told me I had walking pneumonia—the first of five times I'd be diagnosed with this over the next two decades.

Although I soon got over Lisa Kulaska, the same couldn't be said for gambling. I continued to bet and lose increasingly large amounts of money I didn't have. And there was nothing that was too asinine to bet on: tetherball, how much strangers weighed, the number of watts in a lightbulb. A few months later, my mother picked up the other phone line and heard me betting on baseball with a bookie. She told me to "stop this nonsense immediately." And I did. Cold turkey. And I never told my dad about how I used his comic book collection to try to feel up a teenage girl in a back brace. Instead, I cut the lawn every week, waxed his car without being asked and have always gotten him really good Father's Day gifts.

Years later, as I drove around my old neighborhood, I'd see that the Feldmans had a new deck, the Bevalaquas a new car and the Kunoffs new aluminum siding. And I wondered how much of that was because the Hendersons insisted to Richard Dawson that a couch *could* fit in a suitcase.

4

LIFTING

I hated being scrawny. I was skinny, in a "you can see the contour of my bones" way. My teenage arms were so thin I never left the house without wearing thick, tight sweatbands on my wrists so they'd squeeze the flesh up into my forearms, giving the illusion I had upgraded to actual arms. Then the summer between seventh and eighth grades things got worse. I shot up from five feet three inches to five feet ten. Now I was *tall* and skinny, which I hated even more because being the tallest kid in school just drew more attention to my skinniness. And besides, Fonzie wasn't tall.

Growing up, *Happy Days* was my favorite TV show. Like Richie Cunningham, Ralph Malph and Potsie Weber, I thought Arthur Fonzarelli was the coolest guy on the planet. I wanted to be exactly like the Fonz and I couldn't do it towering over everyone. I was now just two inches shy of six feet, a very un-Fonzie-esque height.

Every night before I went to bed I prayed to God that I would stop growing. I didn't ask Him for very much. Not only did I have the rabbi abandonment issue but if there was anything I really wanted or needed I'd just ask my parents. But enough was enough. So I prayed that God would give away some of my height to Larry Sadowski. He'd really appreciate it. I even slept curled up in the fetal position in case God needed a visual clue to my needs.

I rationalized that the more I could emulate Fonzie, the safer I would be. And I needed to protect myself. Yes, I know, being a Jew on Long Island wasn't the toughest situation in the world. However, inside my house, life was scary. I feared that my body was vulnerable, not only to internal forces like disease, but to external harm. My grandfather repeatedly told me: "When I was in Poland and the pogroms began, they went around beating up the Jews, but I fought back." At five feet ten, 110 pounds, I didn't think I was capable of fighting back. Hell, Jews weren't exactly renowned for their physical prowess. I was scared. Despite being 5,000 miles and thirty-two years away from Hitler, I needed some help.

Luckily, help was five houses away.

Mr. Wilkington was a low-key, smiley sixty-seven-year-old white-haired Cub Scout leader who lived down the street with his mother. My brother had known him for years from his involvement with the Scouts. I often ran into Mr. Wilkington while walking Rufus past his house. One afternoon he stopped me.

"Hello, Brian. I just got a new weight set for the troops. Would you like the old weight set that your brother donated a few years back?"

I had no idea my brother had lifted a weight in his life.

"Sure, Mr. Wilkington." I smiled.

I dropped Rufus off at home and enthusiastically ran back to reclaim my brother's old weight set.

The collection consisted of a single barbell with about ninety pounds of concrete-filled plastic-coated weights. The red discs weighed twenty-five pounds; the blue, ten; and the white, five. I rolled the barbell down the sidewalk and was exhausted by the time I pushed it into my garage. But something had happened in that hundred yards. My legs ached, my arms had filled with blood and my shoulders became stiff and immobile. I felt awesome!

I started lifting steadily in my garage and before long I was seeing results. My shirts were tighter, my wrists were finally sweatband-free and my chest was catching up to my sister's. And, as my biceps grew, so did my anxiety. All I could think about all day was lifting. As I sat in homeroom, I'd map out each workout in advance and visualize myself going through every movement. I was extra attentive to training all parts of my body equally so I wouldn't be one of those idiots like Gary Goldstein with a huge upper body and chicken legs. I lifted until failure on every set, relishing the burning sensation of my muscles as the lactic acid dripped into my limbs. And to soothe the burning in my left testicle, I took warm baths whenever I could.

I soon owned several dumbbells, an incline bench, a chin-up bar and an additional hundred pounds of weights. The moment I got home from school I would open up the garage door and start lifting. People walking past my house just stared as I grunted. My parents were supportive of my new hobby, probably because it meant I wasn't in the house as much, so they could yell at each other in the presence of fewer witnesses.

People were starting to notice my new physique. Especially me. As I sat in Mr. Blouin's English class, I would wear skintight T-shirts and periodically pump each biceps an identical number of times and then inspect them to make sure they were still approximately the same size.

All the chin-ups began to widen my back, which meant that my arms were no longer pointing straight down like a normal person's. Instead, each hung from my shoulders at forty-five-degree angles, to make it readily apparent to any bystander that I was, in fact, a lifter. Or attempting to impersonate a pyramid.

When I tagged along with my father to strangers' homes to see if any of their old comics were worthy of purchase, they would inevitably make a comment about my body. "Wow, Sam . . . your son has some big arms there."

"Now if only he could develop his mind," my father would reply in his cadence-free manner.

One day as I was walking home from the bus stop with my new monkeylike gait, Mr. Wilkington stopped me.

"Hello, Brian!" he said as he checked me out. "I can't believe how much progress you've made."

"Thanks!" I said as I flexed my arms in hopes of additional compliments.

"You should come over sometime so I can take your measurements."

"Uh . . . sure . . . sounds good."

I don't want to use the excuse of this sounding creepy in hindsight. Even back then I knew there was something inherently wrong with the scenario. I apprehensively walked down into Mr. Wilkington's basement, which was the messiest room I had ever seen in my life. Papers were strewn everywhere and the scattered Boy Scout memorabilia made it look as if a library had been ransacked by a bunch of Vikings who'd left behind their merit badges.

Mr. Wilkington had stacks and stacks of loose-leaf binders all filled with Polaroid photos of young boys flexing. Below each photo he'd written the date the picture was taken so progress could be charted. He flipped through several of the books to show me the dramatic growth of dozens of boys while narrating each of their backstories.

"Anthony here only weighed one hundred twenty when I met him. Now he's nearly one hundred ninety-five pounds with only eight percent body fat."

"Barry put on thirty-five pounds in a little over a year and can squat over two hundred now!"

"Frederick has a forty-three-inch chest and a twenty-nine-inch waist."

I felt inadequate.

As I fixated on other boys' pecs, Mr. Wilkington tapped me on the shoulder. He was holding a cloth tape measure and a yellow legal pad.

"It's time to measure you, Brian," he pronounced, with a glint in his eye.

He proceeded to snugly wrap the tape measure around my biceps, triceps, chest, waist, thighs, neck and calves, meticulously recording the size of each on his pad. Then he had me take off my shirt and flex while he took several Polaroids. I felt self-conscious and awkward but did as I was told. Frederick, Barry and Anthony had obeyed.

"You'll come back in a couple of months and we'll see how you've grown!"

Sounds good, old creepy guy.

I put myself on a program I read about in Arnold Schwarzenegger's *Encyclopedia of Bodybuilding,* which incidentally weighed nearly thirty pounds. It was a workout just to carry it out of the bookstore. That Arnold was a genius. It's still hard to believe that as a teenager, he was my favorite author.

Throughout high school I kept buying more and more equipment, lifting and reading about lifting in my dank garage. I became so goal-obsessed, I felt that any day I didn't get bigger was a wasted day. I needed those endorphins flowing through my bloodstream or I felt like a deflated loser.

By my senior year I weighed close to 170 pounds and could bench-press nearly 260. And, because my pro-Fonzie prayers had been answered, I was still the five feet ten I had been five years earlier. However, the rest of my body had grown. Thanks to Mr. Wilkington's meticulous records, my biceps had gone from thirteen inches to nearly seventeen, my chest from thirty-three inches to forty, and my quads from twenty-two inches to twenty-seven. According to Arnold's encyclopedia, one's biceps, calves and neck were supposed to be the exact same size, so I became fixated with keeping the three in proportion. I think even Mr. Wilkington appreciated my attention to detail, perhaps more so when I wasn't around.

My penchant for lifting got even more intense in college. While all the freshmen at Emerson were drinking, fucking, joining fraternities and experiencing the euphoria of being away from their parents for the first time, all I did was lift. I rarely went to parties, bars or anywhere that didn't have a squat rack. I couldn't help it. I was an iron junkie, addicted to barbells.

I woke up at five-thirty every morning so I could lift for two hours before my eight o'clock classes. And I made sure I got to bed by ten so I could get my seven and a half hours' sleep. If I didn't, I felt that my subsequent workout was doomed. Although I could see improvements on a weekly basis, I was never satisfied. I had officially become a prisoner of my body, although my captivity was voluntary.

During Christmas break, I was back on Long Island doing one-armed chin-ups in the hallway outside my bedroom when I overheard my parents discussing someone named "Andrew." At first I just assumed it was one of my father's unruly first-graders. With my ear pressed up against their bedroom door, I continued to hear them speak in hushed tones. But why were they whispering? What was so important about this "Andrew" fellow? I knocked on the door. The whispering turned to silence. I was onto something!

"What is it?" came a voice from the other side.

"It's me."

"Yes?"

"Can I come in?"

The answer wasn't always yes. We had many a conversation through wood. My mother's door was practically always locked, as was the hallway bathroom, which was also connected to her bedroom via a second door. Unfortunately, in addition to my mother's other ills, she also had a bad stomach and would never be able to make it to the other bathroom downstairs in time should the upstairs one be occupied. Since the downstairs bathroom consisted of a sink and toilet but no bath or shower, we would have to check in advance with her to make sure "it was a good time." So we often left for school without our maximum cleanliness potential—which bothered all of us except my father.

This time, however, my dad turned the inside knob to let me in.

"What is it?"

"Who's Andrew?"

"That's none of your concern," droned my father.

Secrets were nothing new for my family. No one gave up information unless pummeled by questions or badgered incessantly.

"C'mon! Just tell me who he is. He must be important since you're whispering about him."

"He *is* important, Brian," my mother finally relented. "He's your brother."

"I have a brother named Andrew? Wow!"

"He's dead."

Talk about a buzzkill.

"You never knew about Andrew because he died before you were born," she relayed.

"How did he die? Why didn't you tell me? What was he like?" I had hundreds of questions I wanted answered immediately.

"He was only seven months old when he died."

"Oh my God! What happened?!"

"SIDS."

"Oh. SIDS!" I had absolutely no idea what SIDS was, but I figured I could look it up in the *World Book* later.

"Sudden infant death syndrome," my mother explained. "He died in his sleep."

My parents had only one picture of him. It was a black-and-white Polaroid and he had dark hair and dark eyes and looked more like my mother and brother than my father, sisters and me. He wore a sad expression on his face, as if he knew he wouldn't be around very long.

I soon learned that when Andrew was born, one of my mother's brothers, who had a warped sense of humor, sent her a sympathy card as a joke. This infuriated my mother while Andrew was alive, but became even more distasteful after he was buried. My mother and uncle then took a thirty-eight-and-a-half-year hiatus from speaking due to the misappropriation of a Hallmark product.

"When did he die?"

"About ten months before you were born."

"So you guys actually had five kids. Wow! That's a lot for Jews."

"Actually"—my mother sighed—"had Andrew lived, we wouldn't have had you."

At that very moment, my entire perspective on life shifted. Not only could I potentially get sick as abruptly as my mother, I could die just as suddenly as Andrew. I was already a frenzied and frantic adolescent, but from that day I learned I was a replacement baby, I turned it up a notch and resolved to accomplish as much as I could as quickly as humanly possible before my time was up. Every hour would be rush hour.

First thing on the agenda: bodybuilding competitions.

I mailed in my application and entry fee for Mr. Natural New England as a college sophomore. For a mere $40, the president of the American Natural Bodybuilding Conference would allow me to stand on a stage in a tiny Speedo and show strangers my six-pack, which I thought was a bargain.

For bodybuilding novices, "natural" means steroid-free. A lot of my friends at the gym were taking steroids, but I never even considered it. I had witnessed too many guys who had stopped taking them fall into deep depressions because they couldn't bench-press as much as they used to. Plus, I didn't want to feel paranoid and attribute internal pains when I was fifty to some non-FDA-approved shortcut drug I took in my twenties. I had enough anxiety as it was.

My pre-competition training regimen turned out to be tougher than anything I'd ever done. In addition to lifting weights for two hours a day, I also had to lie in a tanning bed for an hour to toast my pasty-white skin—so that spectators could see the separations between my muscles more easily. For another hour a day, I practiced flexing and holding each pose while maintaining a cheesy smile that told the world that this was effortless.

Like it's normal for a human being to show off the width of his back. I even hired a ballet instructor to help me with my transitions between poses and would awake at four-thirty in the morning for our five o'clock sessions. Not only was bodybuilding getting expensive, but what idiot in college gets up less than three hours after Letterman ends so he can flex his calves?

And then there's the eating. Perhaps the worst pitfall in bodybuilding, something that I still battle with, is the feeling that if I'm not perpetually stuffing my face, my muscles will wither away. Calories were stocked as if my body was a Costco warehouse. If I didn't eat something every two hours, I'd freak and swear that a biceps or quad was deflating. An ex-girlfriend informed me that I had "Bigarexia."[2]

I was obsessed with keeping my body weight as high as possible. Protein became my best friend. I would eat to maximum capacity every few hours. Seven days a week. Month after month after month. And fuck the cardio. That would burn too many calories and make my muscles long and lean—the antithesis of my life's new ambition.

I became so leery of "wasting calories" that I'd wait three hours for my roommates to come home to bring up the mail, rather than squander a precious trip down a flight of stairs. Every ounce of my energy was saved for cosmetic purposes.

On the rare occasions when I would do anything that could, God forbid, actually *stretch* a muscle—like shoot a basketball— I would immediately do an extra session of eating and lifting to return my body to its now permanent contracted state. I became so fanatical that even when I spent a semester abroad in Robertsau, France, I'd travel over an hour a day each way just to get to a gym. The extent of my cross-cultural experience was converting pounds into kilograms.

During the last seven or eight weeks before the competition, I wrote down everything I ate in a notebook and would add up

2. Bigarexia is ostensibly the opposite of anorexia, the latter of which my friend Josh, who knows every doctor in town, has but won't admit.

each day's caloric intake. Banana: 100; Orange: 65; Can of tuna in water: 175; Milk shake: 1,650. Abnormally large banana: 130 (estimated). I would pace myself for a minimum of 6,000 calories a day. But as the competition drew closer, I had to gradually taper off, to whittle away every ounce of fat. And the last week was killer: 800 calories a day. Total. While still working out for two hours. And taking sixteen college credits.

The big day finally arrived. The Huntington, Long Island, auditorium was packed with five hundred fans who had eagerly paid $10 to see striations in men's quads. I was glad I'd told my friends not to come. I didn't need the extra pressure, although there was nobody around anyway. They were all in Fort Lauderdale on spring break like normal college sophomores.

I felt like shit. My muscles were exhausted. My brain was fried. My stomach was the size of a walnut (38 calories). I looked better than I ever had, but was probably less healthy at that moment than the fat guy dry-mopping the stage.

The other bodybuilders were all in the back room, doing push-ups to inflate their muscles and having their pals coat their bodies with baby oil—as you can imagine, an intense and not particularly friendly group of people. But I was too caught up in myself to really care. Besides, I was one of them.

Even under optimum circumstances, there usually wasn't a lot of chatter between bodybuilders. Occasionally, I'd run into a friend from the gym on the street and, no matter who it was, this is pretty much the entire conversation:

"What are you training today?"

"Back and shoulders."

"I'm doing tris and quads."

"Well . . . lemme know if you need a spot."

"'Kay."

They called my group out onto the stage and the flashbulbs in the audience flickered. I was standing in my red Speedo with the number 13 safety-pinned to my hip, sandwiched between some guy named Jordan, who probably weighed close to forty pounds more than me, and someone named Dan who had killer abs but no discernible chest.

The judges bleated out poses and all of us simultaneously flexed the appropriate muscles. The double-biceps flex. The left quad flex. The right triceps flex. Applause erupted for each pose.

While onstage battling hunger and guys with better tans, it hit me. Other men were judging my body. And I was letting them. And I had that dumb "This is effortless" smile on my face the whole time and I thought, "I am so fucking gay right now I cannot stand it."

But I had worked too hard to walk away and I wasn't going to wilt under those 3,000-watt klieg lights. Besides, I had just noticed that both Jordan and Dan were starting to tire. I thought I had a chance. I decided to put all my pain and discomfort on pause. I had worked too hard to get to this point, and I could always go to therapy later to figure out why I was doing this. Right now, it was time to kick some bodybuilding ass. I unleashed my phony smile as I displayed as many veins as possible while simultaneously squeezing my pecs together and expanding my back.

As the judges prepared to announce the winners, I assumed I had finished third or fourth. I thought I had dieted a little too much and had become too lean for my own good. Plus, I didn't have throngs of worshippers with signs shouting out my name and quite possibly bribing the judges with amino acids and protein shakes. The results poured in over a very loud loudspeaker. In third place . . . I can't remember . . . it was a long time ago. In second place . . . still have no idea . . . I'm not great with names of men in Speedos. When they announced that I had finished first, I was in shock. I was Mr. Natural New England 1984. Tall division. I won a large trophy the size of Erin Moran.

However, victory would soon turn to defeat.

Since I had barely eaten over the past few weeks I was literally starving. Luckily, it was time to celebrate. So off I went, by myself, for a post-competition meal to that Mecca of health: IHOP. There my trophy and I ordered a large plate of pancakes, which I wolfed down before the maple syrup had even hit the sides. But I wasn't through. I was craving pizza like a picnic ant. So I went across the street and proceeded to eat an entire pie. Eight slices. In about ten minutes. All by myself.

As the last remnants of crust slid down my throat, I came to a startling conclusion. I didn't feel well. My stomach was killing me. Of course it was! I had gone from 800 calories a day for the past two weeks to 800 calories a minute. I was a moron and my digestive system was in shock.

After a difficult drive back to my parents' house, I staggered inside holding my trophy and they bombarded me with questions about the contest. My mother released the biggest smile I had seen since she took care of me when I had chicken pox. My father insisted I wear his Superman ring for the rest of the week. I just wanted to lie down. But my stomach wouldn't let me. When I couldn't even make it up the stairs to my bedroom, my dad drove me to the hospital.

A doctor informed me that I had eaten so much food that my exponentially expanding stomach had gone through a part of my diaphragm wall. I was diagnosed with a hiatal hernia. I faced potential surgery. In the meantime the gastroenterologist ordered me to have the head of my bed raised to prevent acid from going into my esophagus during the night. Oh, and not to eat *anything,* not even a rice cake. Arnold never mentioned this in his encyclopedia. Thankfully, nearly three days later, after fasting like a Falun Gong leader and letting some 19,000 or so calories take a trip through my intestines, I felt much better.

And I had learned a valuable lesson. Bodybuilding was stupid. And, in hindsight, not exactly a path to calmness. I was tightly wound to begin with; now I was tightly wound with a collection of interminably contracted muscles. Besides, it was time-consuming, expensive and destructive to the mind, skin and internal organs. The pinnacle of pointless self-absorption.

On the other hand, the Mr. Southern Connecticut competition was coming up in April.

And the more trophies I won, the more likely the Nazis would skip over our house and head for the Scheinermanns next door. Now *they* were skinny.

SWALLOWING

The one thing Jews and bodybuilders have in common: we love our food. So when I got that knock on my dorm door, just two months after starting my freshman year of college, I wasn't surprised. Bobby Zellers was looking for someone to represent our floor in the Häagen-Dazs ice cream eating contest at the student center. His first stop was my room.

Although I was by no means a large person, when it came to food I was an absolute animal. And it wasn't just prepping for bodybuilding competitions that made me a savage. I was one way before I ever touched a barbell. Because of my mother's illness, all of my adolescent meals were initiated by the following conversation.

"What do you want tonight? McDonald's, Arby's or Kentucky Fried Chicken?"

"McDonald's."

"Two Big Macs, large fries and a strawberry shake?"

"Yeah. Thanks, Dad."

Not only did my father have to continue teaching first grade and take care of four children and my mother, he was also a full-time waiter.

The other kids in my neighborhood had a different routine. At a preordained time each night, they'd rush home so they could sit around a table with their families to discuss their lives as they ate delicious home-cooked meals. What losers! *My* dad came home from work, took our orders and forty-five minutes later we'd be handed a paper bag with our burgers, drumsticks or roast beef sandwiches. Then off we'd go to our respective rooms to sit alone in front of our respective ten-inch black-and-white TV sets and chow down. No forks, no knives, and often the only napkins would be what we were wearing. We didn't even use spoons for our occasional soup—instead we just tipped the bowl backward and funneled the broth down our throats. I didn't think of us as barbarians; we were just cutting out the cutlery middleman.

The only time we ever sat down and ate together as a family was on Thanksgiving. My dad and I would drive down and pick up a precooked turkey and stuffing from Zorn's, which not only had live turkeys roaming around in the gated area out back but had live peacocks as well—but not to eat, apparently just to make the turkeys feel less attractive.

We'd then pick out some premade stuffing and a prekilled turkey and warm them up in our preheated oven, which was so seldom used we could have just left the door open and let my little sister use it as a desk. Regardless of our diligent preparation, we never made it through the entire meal intact.

Family dining was like playing the game Ker-Plunk: a group of marbles are supported by a series of plastic sticks inserted into a clear Lucite tower. Each player then removes one of the sticks in the hope that it won't be the one to send all of the marbles spiraling to their deaths like a group of handcuffed lemmings. No matter how carefully we watched our words or actions, one of us would invariably end the game of dinner by saying or doing the wrong thing.

"Brian, leave all of the dark meat for your mother, please."

"There's plenty here. She's not going to eat all of it."

"I asked you to *please* leave it!"

"Forget it, Sam!"

Ker-plunk!

Then my mother would storm off and go hobbling upstairs, which would take quite a while and give us plenty of time to try to persuade her to return to the table.

"Ma, come sit down! I put all the dark meat back!"

"Mom! We never get to eat together! Mark drove all the way from Oswego for this!"

"Maw, cool yer pitz and sit back down!"

But our fake peals of protest were ignored. The meal as we knew it was over and we'd have to wait another twelve months for our next food reunion. Anyone who was still hungry would finish in the privacy of his or her own bedroom while watching Tim Conway and Harvey Korman giggle on *The Carol Burnett Show.*

Basically, those truncated Thanksgiving Day meals were the only non-fast-food meals in our house. Which explains my seamless transition into the world of college cafeteria cuisine. While all the other freshmen were incessantly bitching about the food being unhealthy and bland, not only was I pleased with the quality, I was ecstatic about the quantity. It was a veritable two-semester all-you-can-eat buffet.

For me, the Emerson College cafeteria was the happiest place on earth. And I was all for taking advantage of the system. I'd get a large plate of eggplant parmesan, rice and potatoes and then tear into it with the planet's oldest utensils: my hands.

I had no idea this was odd. I thought other students were staring at me because they were just looking around and randomly stopping their eyes at each eater. Instead, they were enjoying the spectacle of my prehistoric dining methods as I violently tore apart food with my fingers. I later learned that the speed at which I ate was astonishing, too. I could go through three plates of food before people sitting near me had even finished one. On the rare occasion that someone would be dumb enough to split an off-campus pizza with me, they'd quickly regret it. They'd be lucky to finish their second slice before the rest of the pie was nestled in my stomach.

My college peers thought I'd been raised by wolverines. Or badgers. Or some other animal that had no concept of how to hold a fork, which to this day is still a little awkward for me. I suppose my parents had far bigger problems than worrying about eating etiquette.

I had unknowingly become a sideshow attraction. After polishing off my entrée, I would trudge over to the ice cream tub for dessert and, without thinking, pile six or seven scoops onto a sugar cone that certainly wasn't built for all that extra weight. I had no idea this was unusual, despite the fact that I was carrying a cone of 10,000 calories which I either needed to hold down by my waist or tilt my head skyward to lick. Then there'd be a race against time before all the Rocky Road or Caramel Swirl would drip through the point of the sugar cone onto the ground. Time usually lost. I wish I'd just been showing off. That would have been a much easier habit to break.

With all the shit I was pouring into my body, it was a miracle I wasn't getting fat along with all the other freshmen. I guess lifting barbells for two hours every day plus a fast metabolism offsets a lot of power eating.

So when Bobby Zellers asked me to represent the sixth floor of our dorm for the Häagen-Dazs contest I was elated. More free food? I'm there! And the best part, with the calorie-whittling phase of the New York Metropolitan bodybuilding competition still months away, I was free to pound down whatever I wanted.

The competition took place in the student center and the place was packed tighter than a quart of Baskin Robbins Nutty Coconut. There were a dozen of us seated behind a pair of really long folding card tables adorned in our complimentary red, one-size-fits-all Häagen-Dazs T-shirts.

I was dwarfed by the other competitors and felt like a featherweight in a heavyweight bout. Tommy Murran was the favorite. He weighed nearly three hundred pounds and his mouth was so large it looked as if he could have swallowed a pumpkin whole. Warren Henneman was also expected to be a dairy conqueror. He tipped the scales at about 225, played center for the college basketball team and was extremely athletic. Frankly, I couldn't have cared less who won as long as I got to eat free ice cream for the next fifteen minutes.

The rules were simple. Eat as much Häagen-Dazs as possible really really fast. Which was pretty much what I'd been doing my entire life—only not on a stage.

The Häagen-Dazs representative blew a whistle and the contest began. For the next quarter of an hour a dozen non-lactose-intolerant students would be eating cold stuff. I had a little advantage. While everyone else was struggling with a variety of spoons and scoopers, I dug my fleshy claws in and scooped out fistfuls of ice cream. No need for teaspoons and tablespoons when you have handspoons.

A switch in my head went off and I was like a South African diamond miner tunneling into pint after pint of Häagen-Dazs. I went through my first container in a little over two minutes while Tommy Murran was barely halfway through his.

The shocked Häagen-Dazs rep immediately placed pint number two in front of me and I attacked it with a vengeance. Warren Henneman was trying to be way too neat, as if he were eating in front of the Queen. It's a competition about eating, not etiquette, schmuck!!! However, there would be no trash-talking, since all of our mouths were occupied.

I breezed into my third pint. Everyone else remained on his first. My chunky competitors were quickly being left in the dust.

"Gimme another pint, Ice Cream Man!!!!" I mumbled as I discarded my most recently devoured container onto the ground.

Ten minutes into the competition, I had finished nearly four pints. As I continued to scoff down my Fudge Swirl, I realized several things. One: I should have brought mittens. My hands were freezing. It felt as if I had been in a snowball fight for the last three days. Two: my teeth, tongue, palate and throat were starting to get uncomfortable, as if a glacier was passing through my esophagus. Three: when does the hot apple pie competition start, 'cause this is starting to blow?

As my entourage of ice cream merged down my larynx, my brain finally sent a message down to my mouth to close up shop. I couldn't finish the contest. And it had nothing to do with my stomach being full.

My entire head felt like an ice sculpture and my fingers were totally numb. But in the scant twelve minutes I'd been eating frozen stuff, I had managed to quaff down a school record four and a half pints. Unless one of the other contestants could eat an unlikely pint a minute, this thing was in the bag. And both Tommy Murran and Warren Henneman looked nauseated.

I sat and watched the final three minutes with a giant headache, wishing I had been born wearing a parka.

When the lactose settled, I had won handily. As the crowd cheered my gluttony, I felt like Nixon in '72, squashing a squadron of McGoverns. Then the proud Häagen-Dazs representative stepped onto the stage and awarded me my prize: a certificate for a free scoop of Häagen-Dazs for everyone on my dorm floor. Huh? That's it? No giant cone-shaped trophy? No silo of sprinkles? No entry into the Ice Cream Hall of Fame? I hated this contest! I had risked my life and extremities for my fellow students and all I got was the equivalent of $1.50, which, even back in the early '80s, sucked.

There were no high fives exchanged that day. An hour later, my hands were still so numb I had trouble unlocking my dorm room door. And forget about flossing. I woke up the next morning and although my fingers had thawed, my mouth was still throbbing. There was no way I could make my History of TV class that day.

I went to the school infirmary and told the doctor what happened. Hi, I'm the idiot who ate five pints of ice cream in ten minutes so my friends could all get free sugar cones. Li'l help?

The doctor examined my mouth and informed me that I had frostbite. I thought only Eskimos, Iditarod mushers and Clarence Birdseye got frostbite—not college freshmen seated at folding tables in heated ballrooms in October. I was instructed to gargle with warm cider vinegar for three weeks and stay away from cold things. But, as always, now that I had a diagnosis and a solution, I was pleased: committed to healing yet another self-inflicted wound.

For the better part of the next month, I drove my roommate (and me) crazy with the acrid odor of the cider vinegar and my perpetual gargling sessions. Unlike whistling, gargling is one of the few noises that annoys even the person doing it. I reminded my cohabitant that this was the price he had to pay for the free scoop of pistachio I had scored him. Now put the cap back on the toothpaste, you cretin!

About a month later, my face finally felt like my face. And despite all the ice cream trauma, I was soon back in the cafeteria stuffing myself and arguing with everyone that college food really *was* delicious.

6

(Not) Chewing

I started doing stand-up in college. I had stumbled into the profession when a Comedy Writing professor at Emerson required that everyone perform five minutes for the class at the end of the semester. My first joke was semi-melodically singing, "What would you think if I sang outta key?" and then a key, which I'd hidden under my tongue before class, would fall to the ground after I'd spit it out. For whatever reason, that was the beginning of a new career, enabling me to quit my night job at Marlboro Market walking through aisles, pulling items on shelves forward.

For the better part of the next ten years, I continued to pursue both bodybuilding and stand-up. Just as I didn't reveal my personality in bodybuilding, I didn't want to reveal anything about my body in comedy clubs. So my gym friends had no idea I did stand-up (laughing and hack squats don't mix), and my comedy friends had no clue I lifted weights (I wore really baggy clothes so they wouldn't mock me).

Besides, I didn't want my trapezoids distracting from what I was saying. Not that what I was saying was very important. Basically, I yelled all my jokes as veins popped out of my neck like a series of suspension bridges and my face turned beet red, giving little insight into myself besides being pretty angry. A Boston newspaper referred to me as "a glue-sniffing Doberman," which may have been an understatement.

My mother was interested in both of my pursuits. She carried a picture in her purse of me flexing in a Speedo and showed it to her various doctors, whether or not they were interested. She also became a connoisseur of comedy, following my stand-up peers on television as they made it big. And her critiques were scathing. She was more jealous of them than I was. But at least I had a fan.

At twenty-eight, I moved my stand-up act to Manhattan so I could be heckled by people with New York accents. There, the years of Bigarexia bingeing caught up to me. Several times a month my colon would randomly pulsate and contract, followed by a few short bursts of acute, searing pain. Two years prior, my colon had hemorrhaged and I was rushed to the hospital, where I spent the next three days hooked up to an IV to replenish the fluids my body had emptied. I'd lost so much blood and was so dehydrated the nurse couldn't even find a vein to stick the tube in. I had colitis. When the doctor asked if I was under a lot of stress, I answered, "Not that I know of." But in retrospect, the more accurate reply would have been, "Yes, but only for the past fifteen or sixteen years, sir."

Like many Manhattanites, my living conditions were less than ideal. I shared a one-bedroom apartment in the West Village with a sixty-eight-year-old man who sang opera at four in the morning and would disappear for a week at a time, leaving me to clean up a week of his Australian shepherd's shit in the living room. It was bad enough I had to monitor a strange dog's colon; I wanted mine to be trouble-free. I thumbed through the yellow pages and found a place on the Lower East Side that specialized in this sort of thing.

A bright-eyed, cheery Scandinavian-looking woman named Gretchen, who was a little too fond of eyeliner, greeted me at the door.

"Hi, are you here for a monthly cleaning?"

"Monthly? People have this done once a month?"

"Healthy people do."

I wrote out a check for $54 and put on a sea-foam green paper hospital dress with an open back for easy access. I was instructed to lie flat, facedown on a padded gray table. Then, without a moment's notice, Gretchen shoved $54 worth of rubber hose up my ass. It completely startled me. I was expecting some small talk first, as most doctors attempted when they were taking blood or giving me my allergy shots.

"Say, Brian, pretty hot out today, huh?"

Then jab! While I was thinking about the question, a needle would puncture my arm. I'm sure doctors giving death-row inmates lethal injections have better bedside manner than Gretchen.

This invasive process was followed by gallon after gallon of water being pumped through the hose into my intestines. After what felt like enough fluid to sail a boat on was in me, I was told to prop up my upper body to a forty-five-degree angle so everything could drain. As I did so, Gretchen wedged a small plastic container under my non-face cheeks as various "materials" came racing out of my system.

"Oh, no!"

"Oh, no, what?" I trembled.

"I've never seen anything like this!"

"Like *what*? I've got a tube stuck in my ass! Can you please try not to scare me?!"

"You don't chew your food."

"Of course I chew my food."

"You don't chew it enough! There are *huge* chunks of unchewed food in your system. You really need to do something about this. It's pretty serious."

I instantly sweated through my paper gown and began to have an anxiety attack. My pulse raced, my breath shortened, my face turned white, my vision blurred, I got dizzy and nearly blacked out. I didn't chew my food! It was so fucking simple to chew food. Damn it! Another set of internal organs ruined! For all the weights I was lifting and all the drugs and alcohol I was avoiding and as good as I was at staying away from my childhood friends fried food and junk food, my haste in everything I did was coming back to haunt me.

"Are you okay?"

"Yeah . . . I'll be all right . . . I just need to lie down on a cold floor. Is there any linoleum here?"

Gretchen escorted me to the bathroom, where I remained prone for about fifteen minutes, breathing deeply.

"Should I call a doctor?"

"No. I'll be fine. Really. Just some more deep breaths and I'll be back to normal."

After I returned to my upright self, I asked Gretchen what I should do.

"Well, you obviously have some issues with food . . ."

"Among other things," I chimed in, trying to make the ass lady grin.

"I think you should see Irene. I'll write down her number for you. She's a food coach."

A food coach? What the hell was a food coach? Were there whistles and yelling involved? I had to try it.

Irene Robbins was an ultra-serious, fortysomething, dark-haired, overly skinny woman who looked like she had either the world's healthiest skin or a really shitty fake tan. After a brief introduction I was motioned to have a seat across from her maple desk in her swank Upper East Side office. As I sat down, I saw it! And I began to squirm in my seat and get dizzy, again approaching Blackout Land. Irene eyeballed my convulsive actions in confusion but said nothing.

"Can you . . . uh . . . this is gonna sound REALLY insane . . . but can you put that glass of milk somewhere other than right in my line of vision?"

"The milk?" she asked incredulously. "The *milk* is bothering you?"

"Actually I would say it's more like it's taunting me, but bothering works, too."

I hadn't had a glass of milk since I was six months old. My mother said that when the nipple on the bottle I was being fed with broke, I just stopped drinking it. My parents, grandparents, aunts and uncles then tried to force-feed me milk, experimenting with an assortment of new nipples on an assortment of new bottles, even trying different types of milk such as goat's and yak's. But my little baby brain wouldn't budge. After just half a year of existence, I had unequivocally ended my relationship with that purest of white substances.

"What about milk shakes?"

"Sure, I've had milk shakes but always of the non-white variety. Can't do vanilla. Only chocolate, strawberry, coffee. And I can't watch when they pour the milk in the blender."

Irene scribbled something in her notebook, which could very well have been, *Must find job where I don't have to work with crazy people.*

"And what happened when you were growing up if someone at your lunch table in elementary school had milk?" she continued.

"I'd change tables."

"You'd get up and change tables?"

"Yes."

"But didn't every child in elementary school drink milk?"

"There were assorted juice drinkers, but yeah, I changed tables a lot."

"And why do you think you're afraid of milk?"

I remained silent for a minute, which was unusual for me.

"I guess because I feel guilt over having messed up the milk-collecting stage of my life and now my bones aren't as strong as other people's."

"So all of this is about guilt?"

"Yeah. Now if there's any structural weakness in my body, it's my fault."

Even today, despite all of my travails, despite being in my forties and on Zoloft, I'm still unable to watch another human drink a glass of milk. Which might also explain why I'm extra terrified to have a kid. The mere sight of white liquid in a bottle would probably make me faint. The only white substance I seem to be able to interact with is Wite-Out.

"Do you have any other food fears?" asked Irene, who didn't bother looking up from her already ink-filled pad.

"Not really . . . Okay, I hate baked beans. I don't know why. I've just always hated them. I hate the smell, I hate the shape, I hate the color. But especially the smell."

"Did you ever have a bad experience with beans?"

"Just watching my father eat them."

I don't mean to imply that he would eat a few and then throw the rest at me. He was more mature than that. My dad would simply sit at the far end of our long, rectangular Formica kitchen table hunched over the bowl like a vulture while he read the newspaper and chomped on them. If I happened to venture into the kitchen for a snack while the bean-eating was taking place, I'd sit at the far end of the table to put maximum distance between me and my brown gooey enemies. But that wasn't enough. The smell would permeate throughout the room and, out of my peripheral vision, I could still see the beans.

"So did you leave?"

"No. I rigged up a handkerchief around the right brim of my Mets hat which formed a mini-scaffolding to shield my eyes from the beans."

"You ate with a handkerchief attached to your hat?"

"Yeah. And once in a while pinching my nostrils, to block out the smell. Sometimes I even ate with nose plugs."

"Did your parents try to break this fear?"

"I think they thought I'd grow out of it."

Irene made more notes.

"What else are you afraid of?"

"Raisins."

I can't stand raisins. Their shriveled-up charcoal mass nauseates me. Yes, I know that raisins come from grapes and, yes, I do drink wine, but it's not the same. I ate one raisin when I was three and the awful taste seemed to spread into every artery within seconds, making my entire body feel polluted and ill. It doesn't help that they look like mouse shit—which comes from mice—another irrational fear passed down to me by my father. In fact, the mere sight of a factory-sealed box of raisins is enough to make each of my intestines convulse. If I'm in a supermarket, I can't even make eye contact with that smirking raisiny woman with the red bonnet on the front of the red box. It's as if she's an ex-girlfriend to whom I owe money and I'd rather eat mouse shit.

"Do you think this is related to the baked beans?"

"Not sure."

"I mean, they're both roughly the same shape. And size."

"That's exactly what my mother has said. I think the baked beans are more of a smell thing and the raisins are more of an aesthetic mishap."

Despite food quirks being her area of expertise, Irene offered no solutions for any of my woes. But she had written a lot of stuff on her pad.

"Okay." Irene sighed. "What I think we should do for next time . . ."

Next time? How could she be so certain that there would even be a "next time"? I mean, she hadn't exactly unlocked the secrets behind my problems. All she did was ask some innocuous questions like an inquisitive waitress.

". . . is meet at a restaurant. So I can take some notes on how you eat."

This made sense. Irene was smart.

A week later we met at a local diner in a booth near the back. Irene now had a small tape recorder and a fancy pen. When the waiter appeared I ordered a chicken breast with rice and broccoli and a large orange juice. I expected Irene to ask for a vanilla milk shake with a scoop of rum raisin ice cream and a side of beans just to torment me. But she ordered exactly what I did, either to kiss my ass or to make it easy to split the bill.

As soon as our food arrived, I began to eat as I normally would. Quickly.

"Ah ah ah!!!" Irene waved her hands around frantically, seconds after my fork left my mouth.

"What?"

"What's the rush?"

"I want to eat my food. It smells good."

"But there's no need to do it *so quickly.* Like Gretchen told you, not chewing your food enough puts undue stress on your internal organs. You want to make sure the work is done up *here*"—she pointed to her mouth overdramatically, like a model on a game show illustrating a speedboat—"and *not* down *here!*"—and with a sweeping arc, her hand patted her stomach.

"Sorry."

"Don't apologize to me. Apologize to your body."

"Sorry, body."

"Why do you rush through your meals like this?"

The truth was, one of the main symptoms of hyper-chondria is never living in the moment. I was always at least one step ahead of whatever I was doing. Unlike my brother and parents, I had no use for nostalgia. The only place I wanted to be was the future. The only trouble was, by the time I got there, it wasn't the future anymore. Patience isn't a side effect of my affliction. Unless I'm waiting to heal.

"I rush through everything, I guess."

I couldn't even leave any food in my refrigerator. Nothing. I've even tasted baking soda from the Arm & Hammer box. Actually, the only reason I even needed a fridge was for ice. If I went shopping, whether for a can of soup or $75 worth of groceries for the week, it would all be gone before I went to sleep. All of it. I couldn't control myself. My method of dealing was simple: whenever I was hungry I'd go out and get only enough food for a single meal.

I'd learned to eat quickly from my dad. On the rare occasions that I saw him with food, his goal was speed—most likely because his chewing was constantly interrupted by my mother shouting from her bedroom, needing help.

"I want you to try something for me. For a week." Irene took a sip of her juice for emphasis. "You can finish your meal here at whatever speed you'd like, but the *second* you leave this diner, I want you to chew every bite forty times."

"Forty times?"

"It just seems like a lot because right now you're chewing everything two or three times, if that. Do you want me to show you photos of the stomachs and intestines of people who under-chew their food?" I still wonder what her reaction would have been had I answered with an enthusiastic "YES! Show me those pictures! Pleeeeeeaaaase?!" Then when she did, I'd stare at them awestruck. "This is soooooo cool! You mean if I keep doing what I'm doing I can have organs like that? Yippee!!!" But I remained silent and let her finish her tirade.

"It's not pretty."

I decided I had nothing to lose. I would make an effort to chew everything extremely thoroughly, as if each and every morsel I thrust into my mouth was a stick of gum—which isn't the best analogy, since I'm incapable of not stuffing the entire pack into my mouth within minutes, even if it contains eighteen pieces. Everything would be chewed forty times and I would be instantly cured. And if my body ever required an autopsy, the coroner would marvel at my pristine inner organs.

I returned home to my empty refrigerator that night and began my new life-enhancing procedure. I ordered in some chicken curry from a local Thai place and turned off the ringer on my phone. This was the night that I would finally taste my food.

I hunkered down above my steaming dinner in Styrofoam. The plastic fork secured a small piece of the curry-soaked chicken which I released into the comfort of my mouth. "Chewing is good," I said to myself. "You're doing an excellent thing for your body. In fact, if stomachs could write, I'd probably get a thank-you card." I chewed for what felt like an hour and had only reached the number seventeen. Yet despite all my efforts and powerful saliva enzymes, the chicken wasn't even fully ground up yet. Even all this chewing wasn't nearly enough. I caught my breath and continued on for what seemed like another hour, until I finally reached the magic number. I stared down at my food, of which 98 percent remained. And I was sad.

Food had always been a source of joy and comfort for me. It took my mind off troubles, it nourished my body, it gave me a popular hobby I could share with others. Now food kind of sucked. All food. I tried a piece of the potato in the potato compartment and got up to the number thirty before I said "Fuck it" and devoured the remainder of the meal in less time than it had taken to down the first two bites. I would start this new chewing system tomorrow. Baby steps.

I walked around Manhattan miserable. I didn't want to have to work so hard for my meals. If I could have carried a blender in my pocket and lived on smoothies I would have, but to my chagrin the smoothie had yet to captivate America.

Overnight, eating was transformed from big fun into a big pain.

But I had to stick to this chewing thing for at least a week, as I promised Irene. One thing I'm good at is following rules from medical professionals. When a dentist recently informed me that I needed to spend four minutes brushing my teeth (two for top, two for bottom), I bought a timer and have diligently continued the process to this day. But chewing was way harder than oral hygiene.

Whenever I had offers from friends to go out to dinner, I declined. I didn't want to let them see me suffer. Or to catch me tapping my foot to count my chews. Eating at home—without witnesses—was painful enough. Each time the fork left my mouth I'd sit on my hands until my chewing regimen had been completed to make sure I didn't shovel an additional bite down my throat. Often, I'd stare at my meal while I was immersed in a morsel and blink very fast so my plate would look empty for part of the time. I was going insane. Chewing was so torturous, I even considered going food shopping and leaving edibles in my refrigerator for a change, since eating everything in it under these rules would take forever and possibly crack my mandible.

At the end of the seven-day experiment, I called Irene and told her how much better I felt. Then I canceled all future appointments with her. Charging $300 for information she could have written on a fortune cookie was wrong. I was on my own now. I could decide how many times things would be chewed. I was again the master of my mouth. I had the power. Maybe I'd chew a cracker twenty-six times but a knish nineteen times. I'd chew a mustard sandwich five times but a burned waffle thirty-nine and a half times. Or to show off, I'd chew a piece of dried apple forty-seven times. I would mix it up as I saw fit. But I would try to slow down.

However, it would be another two bodybuilding competitions, hundreds of doctors' visits, 15,000 partially chewed meals and tens of thousands of unnecessary self-induced moments of tension over the next decade before I really made a concerted effort to get better.

PART TWO

100 mg

7

LAMINATING

Nancy and I had been married for a little over seven blissful months. On any given day, I was calmer than at any other point in my life. My mind and body no longer sabotaged each other like in a Tom and Jerry cartoon, I wasn't getting sick or raising my voice or pointing my fists at strangers, and driving was something I actually looked forward to.

Until the third week of that seventh month when that guy in the Honda cut me off and gave me the finger and I threatened to kill him.

It was apparent that 50 mg of Zoloft would not solve my problem. And 100 wouldn't either. And I'm guessing neither would 150. The trouble is, I'd never know exactly *when* my serotonin would fail to be blocked and sneak back into a nerve cell and I'd be back to square one, having to up my dose yet again. Before I reached the maximum 200 mg, I needed to hurry up and find something that would calm me down naturally.

"I'm getting off the Zoloft," I announced to Nancy.

"Today?"

"No. But I can't keep relying on it. Now that I know how a normal human is supposed to feel and behave, I need to wean myself off this crap and deal with my hyperness without drugs."

"Just make sure you talk to your dermatologist before you do anything. It seems wrong to wean on your own."

"I can wean on my own."

"Please don't. You're not a doctor."

"Neither is a dermatologist, really."

"He's still more of a doctor than you are."

"I don't want to be at the mercy of Pfizer a day longer than I have to. What if a hurricane hits Los Angeles and we're stranded in the middle of nowhere and I don't have my medication?"

"Everyone would be stressed, so you wouldn't really stick out *that* much."

"Well, I'm gonna find Zoloft alternatives that I don't have to swallow."

"As long as you don't yell at me when I drive, I'm totally supportive of anything you do."

"Don't sweat the smawl stuff . . . and it's awwwwlllllll smawlll-lll stuff!" Since Richard Carlson wrote that fateful phrase back in 1997, that sentence has pretty much annulled every problem for my older sister, Debbie. Whether you've just spilled pudding on a shoe, or a shark has eaten the left hemisphere of your brain, my sister consistently applies that magical series of words to put things into perspective.

Debbie has three unruly teenage kids, a husband with myriad health problems and 90 percent of the calls she gets are from people who are dying. She's a hospice nurse in Florida and often our conversations will be interrupted by call-waiting. When she clicks back to me, I'm told the person on the other line was a twelve-year-old boy with leukemia or a nine-year-old girl who has a disease so rare they haven't even named it yet and by the time they do, she'll most likely be dead.

It was Debbie's idea for my parents to move to Florida. This way they could get an affordable one-level house and have the safety net of one of their children nearby. Debbie continues to take on more responsibility, which to me is a recipe for more anxiety. But she seems to manage.

My sister found a house in the newspaper on a Tuesday and told my father about it on a Wednesday; he flew down to Florida on a Thursday, put in a bid for it and flew home on Fri-

day. By Saturday he knew that his entire life was being transferred to Sarasota. Incidentally, in spite of all his fears, my father finds the prospect of bouncing around in a metal tube at
30,000 feet soothing.

Debbie's home is coated in inspirational sayings, which, I
must say, is fairly unusual for Jews. As a group, we're not huge
consumers of calligraphy and probably fall in the lower per-
centiles of pithy sayings in loud, garish frames per capita. But
perhaps Debbie isn't all that Jewish anymore, anyway.

Twenty-four years ago, my sister married Von, a Protestant
whose family wasn't so keen on getting involved with any Jews.
One would have thought that if someone disliked this chunk of
the Judeo-Christian sect so much, then maybe Long Island
wasn't the place to live. In any event, her wedding consisted of
his family on one side of the ballroom floor and ours on the other.
The only mingling was when people spilled things.

The kicker came many years later when Debbie and Von's
eldest son, Doug, was sent to the local Catholic high school.
Needless to say, my parents weren't all too pleased with some
of the curriculum.

"Grandma, so *you* actually believe in God?!" Doug asked.

"Of course we believe in God," my mother replied.

"But how could you if you killed Jesus?!"

Because *God* told us to kill Jesus, ya silly goose!

If Debbie could handle the stresses of taking care of my parents, forty hospice patients, three kids (at least one of whom
had stumbled into anti-Semitism) and a husband whose failing
eyes were making it impossible to drive, then I would give her
method a try. My life was a picnic compared to hers.

I'm usually vehemently opposed to inspirational words. I
find them cheesy. I particularly detest that Robert Fulghum
crap: *All I Really Need to Know I Learned in Kindergarten.* Oh,
really, Robert? You learned how to make pasta in kindergarten?
You learned how to drive a car in kindergarten? You learned
how to pour a Black and Tan in kindergarten? I think you're a
bit of an exaggerator, Robert.

I headed down to Barnes & Noble with a notebook and pencil to scour Anger Management–type books for some memorable quotes. I'm against spending money on books that I'll only need for six or seven words. However, I'm very pro–book buying. I promised myself I'd purchase the new Churchill biography and a fresh Thomas Guide for Nancy on the way out.

While I was weaving around and over squatters seated in aisles reading shit for free, my goal was to refrain from "accidentally" kicking them while gathering as many powerful sentences as I could that would fit on two sides of a small credit-card-sized piece of paper in eight-point Helvetica.

Look forward to difficulties.

Ooh. That was a good one. Plus, it was only four words, so it wouldn't take up much space.

Don't let your mind be a bad bouncer that lets every emotion into your brain.

I liked that one, too. I needed to have my mind cordon off every feeling behind my velvet ropes and let only the coolest and hippest emotions into "Club Brain." Unfortunately, I have this big dumb bouncer standing guard who had to cheat to get a combined 550 on his SATs.[3] In fact, my bouncer is such an idiot that any emotion with a lame fake ID or a nice smile who he thinks might fuck him at the end of the night, or who lies and claims to be an old friend of my cerebellum, is whisked right in. I've tried to fire my bouncer numerous times but he refuses to leave.

Give up the idea that things will be the way you expect.

3. 350 Math, 200 Verbal, totally spaced on the Essay section.

Sure. That makes the card, too. I could always kick this quote off later if something better came along.

After selecting some more collections of anti-anger words, I went home, typed and printed them out, cutting the paper into the same dimensions as my Wells Fargo debit card. I then glued both parts together so I had a two-sided rectangle that would fit in my wallet. The only thing left to do was get it laminated.

When I gave the Kinko's clerk my inspiration cheat sheet, he glanced down at the first few quotes, then back up at me, and emitted a subtle, condescending eye-roll. Hold on a second: You're thirty-two years old and working at *Kinko's,* you don't even have a "manager" badge on and you're judging me?! Maybe he thought I was in some cult or a Christian Scientist or something. Actually, I couldn't be any farther away from Christian Science, which forbids all contact with doctors, whereas my address book had more physicians than friends. I've always found it odd that an entire group of people could be talked out of ever seeing an entirely different group of people. Did Christian Scientists even bother to get medical insurance or were they that confident about being able to heal themselves? And if they got into a car accident, *then* could they go to the doctor or would they just have to pray until all the scars and orbital bones healed?

As I was about to simultaneously give the Kinko's klown $1.20 for my lamination fee and a glare for being a dick, I felt the warmth of the plastic against my hand and I looked down and saw this:

Anger is exaggerating the consequences.

This is a major hurdle for me. The most innocuous of incidents is quickly heightened. A minor, inconsequential event is soon transformed into a full-length feature, which is always, unfortunately, of the horror genre.

Here's what I mean. I'm about to walk into a hardware store. A guy is standing outside in the doorway. He's definitely in the way. Being that I weigh close to 180 pounds, am wearing a loud-patterned shirt and am about a foot away from him *and* in his sight line, it's unlikely that he doesn't see me. Now, the stranger's two choices are to move out of the way so I can go inside and buy some pliers, or not move at all—because maybe, just maybe he has glaucoma and his guide dog just broke free and ran down the street toward the soft pretzel vendor. But instead he sees my walking torso approach and does the unthinkable. He moves approximately *an eighth of an inch*! Now, this effort is absolutely useless to me. An eighth of an inch does me no good at all. But the message is being sent: "Here! I made an effort; this is all the space you deserve! I'm wayyyy more important than you. Go ahead and struggle to squeeze by, asshole!" This guy REALLY doesn't give a shit about my life. In fact, he'd probably ruin every aspect of it if he had the time.

Now, here's where the filmmaking kicks in. Within seconds, I have constructed a series of scenes in my head where I elbow Captain Stationary in the ribs, then kick him in the groin. And while he's writhing in agony on the cold sidewalk, I hold a pair of steak knives *exactly an eighth of an inch* from his eyes. I proceed to his ear area where I yank one off, coat it with honey Dijon mustard and feed it to a nearby squirrel (who will attempt to store it in his cheeks for the entire winter but can't 'cause it's just too goddamn delicious).

But there's plenty of movie left. I stuff the guy into a phone booth as the walls move in until each of the four is *exactly an eighth of an inch* from the other. "Yeah, y'know something . . . you were right, sir. An eighth of an inch is plenty of room to navigate through." I immediately flick a switch and each of the walls moves in so they're one-sixteenth of an inch away from one another and the man's torso is squeezed so tightly his body turns beet red and he looks like a giant Twizzler which I feed to the squirrel's friend who didn't get any ear.

Yes, anger can be full of exaggeration. Irrational? Of course it's irrational. But these are the dots that my brain connects in a millisecond.

Thankfully, I didn't cast the Kinko's guy in my latest homage to *Reservoir Dogs*. Instead, I looked up from my freshly laminated card, smiled and walked out of the copy place with my head held high. I had already gotten my $1.20 worth.

As I drove home I propped the laminated anti-anger card onto the dashboard of my car to remind me that road rage was unwarranted and irrational.

After I had driven all of three blocks, a guy in a charcoal gray Hummer cut in front of me without using his blinker. You'd think people who can afford a $62,000 car have jobs where they're required to retain information on a daily basis and that remembering to use a blinker would be easy for them. Just as I was about to mouth one of my favorite catchphrases, "Asshole!" to him—or her . . . actually, I couldn't see who was driving since most Hummers seem to come with dark tinted glass as a mandatory option—I resisted. Instead, I consulted my laminated card and reread the first quote again:

Anger is exaggerating the consequences.

There was no reason for anger right now. My car hadn't been hit, and I would probably never see the Hummer man or woman again. Besides, my father had always told me that it's better to have crazy drivers in front of you, since they're pretty much harmless that way. In back of you, anything can happen. To this day, if I see somebody swerving, I slow down, let him pass and let other people worry. I concluded that there was nothing to be angry about. Everything was fine.

When I got home I was so excited about my anger-free future that I bragged to Nancy.

"I didn't glare at the guy at Kinko's who rolled his eyes at me and I totally ignored this Hummer that cut me off on the way home!"

I waited for at least a modicum of praise but none came.

"So?"

"So? Isn't that great news?!"

"No. That's *normal* news. That's how people are supposed to behave in society."

It was going to be harder to impress Nancy than I thought.

I shut the bedroom door and Googled "Anger Management" in hopes of gathering up more quotes for a second laminated card. There, in the middle of the first page, I saw something that piqued my interest even more than a series of quotes worthy of draping heated plastic around: an "Understanding and Transforming Anger" course, a mere three highway exits away. The two-part, four-hour program would cost $50, so my anti-anger laminated card and I signed up.

The building was a two-story concrete slab. As usual, I was excessively early. No matter where I was going I was always the first to arrive. Even meeting friends for lunch at a café a mile from my house, I'd arrive at least ten minutes before we had arranged. To me, being on time was being late. My rationale: boredom was a pleasant alternative to a stressful battle with minutes and seconds.

I sat down in the corner of the back row and waited for the other angry people to show up. The advantage of getting somewhere first is that you can avoid getting trapped between two people you'd rather not be near. The wall is your friend and always will be.

I had expected to see a lot of white guys with shaved heads and earrings, most of whom looked as though they had either done jail time or were running late because beating their wives or girlfriends had taken longer than expected. However, the majority of the people drifting in were women. Old women with gray hair and ponytails who looked like they had been waiting on line for Lilith Fair tickets for sixty years;

twentysomething women casually dressed in T-shirts; and women about my age in business suits who had come straight from work.

The room was already a third of the way full and the workshop wasn't going to start for another ten minutes. This turnout had already exceeded my expectations.

There were still at least twenty-five empty chairs when a middle-aged couple came in and sat right next to me, which was uncalled for. There were plenty of other seats that weren't next to anyone! It was as if someone sat next to me on an empty bus. Jerk.

My new neighbor wore a Tommy Bahama shirt with red suede sneakers and had a large William H. Taft–like mustache. I wish I could tell you what his wife looked like, but his giant walrus mustache blocked my view. In any case, he didn't waste a second before he started yapping loudly to her while simultaneously smacking his gum. I considered switching seats, but by the time I had decided to move, there were barely any left.

New stragglers included a couple of guys with shoulder-length hair who looked like either members of bad rock bands or roadies for good ones. A man in a blue pin-striped suit, with a full head of black hair, sat in front of me. He seemed to be a banker, which made sense because people in finance tend to get angry. There always seems to be shouting when lots of money is at stake. I suspected that he had strangled a coworker who had given him a "can't miss" stock tip that quickly did just the opposite. These were not people you wanted to fuck with. I wondered if anybody had been required to enroll as part of a plea bargain or a deal with his or her parole officer.

The instructor walked in at three minutes before the hour. She was a peppy, high-intensity, no-nonsense lady with light red hair, wearing a white sweater with a pink cat on it and was probably on her third face-lift.

"My name is Eileen and I'll be your teacher. This class is sold out, so we'll wait five more minutes for everyone to get here."

It wasn't starting on time! I wondered if this was just a gim-mick to get everyone in class enraged and start a riot and flush out the truly angry. Perhaps there was a bevy of police officers on the other side of the wall, ready to pounce if we acted up.

In the meantime Eileen scribbled "Anger" on a giant flip pad the size of my kitchen table, being sure to make each of the letters really squiggly so the word looked angry. She was one clever lady.

Meanwhile, the gum-snapping next to me continued. It was as if the walrus was popping a giant sheet of bubble wrap in-side his mouth. It was hard to concentrate, even though there wasn't actually anything to concentrate on yet. But if this kept up, I knew it would be hard to concentrate when I had to. The class hadn't even started and I was about to snap. I removed my laminated anger card for a quick consultation.

If there is a remedy and you can repair it, then do it and don't be unhappy; if there isn't a remedy, then there's no point in being unhappy.

Part of the trouble is that I think the second half of the above statement never applies to me. I believe every problem can be "remedied" and fixed. In this instance, I could rip the gum out of Walrus Head's mouth.

I relaxed a little, comforted by my capacity to solve things. Besides, I figured that when the class started, Eileen's resonant, energetic voice would drown out the gum-snapper anyway. I'd have to ride it out. It was too hacky to get angry in Anger Management.

At five after seven, Eileen walked around passing out a packet of articles to each student. Taft turned to his wife and boisterously said, "I didn't study for *this* test!" and then laughed uproariously at his own joke even before he had fin-ished his sentence. I couldn't imagine how loud it would've been had his mustache not absorbed 90 percent of the sound.

"Did you know that when you get angry, the adrenal glands

release cortisol, epinephrine and other stress hormones?" Eileen singsongingly asked. "And then the heart rate speeds up, blood pressure rises and breathing becomes short."

The class seemed to give a collective shrug as if to say, "Yeah, so?"

"Your muscles tense, the brain becomes hyper-alert, while the heart pumps more and more blood to the legs and arms. And that's not all," she said as if she were an electronics salesperson doing an amped-up commercial. "The digestive and immune systems practically *shut down*!"

This was the root of all my hyper-chondria. Being hyped-up, stressed and angry taxed my organs and invited disease into my body. Just what those Australian researchers said in the footnote on page 3.

"But even when you *stop* being angry . . . the stress hormones continue . . . to linger . . . in the bloodstream!" Eileen then repeated it a second time just in case we neglected the importance of her slower cadence. "That's right. Even when you STOP being angry, the stress hormones *continue* to linger in the bloodstream!"

Walrus-mustached Rip Taylor fucker next to me then turned to his wife and jokingly said, "I wish she hadn't told me that: Now I'm even *more* stressed!" Then both of them chortled for what seemed like a minute and a half.

Eileen explained, "Sometimes we just can't seem to escape our rage. But think about this. If a tiger jumped out of that cabinet, you'd forget about your anger, wouldn't you?" That's where she's wrong. I'd be angry at how a tiger got past security and that people didn't spay or neuter their tigers. No matter what, I would find someone or something to blame and get pissed-off at. My anger would be intact. I could logically find anger anywhere.

"But here's some good news." She paused for added emphasis. "Did you know that anger isn't real? Well, it isn't. Anger is always a cover-up for another emotion. That's right! Anger is imaginary. There are a total of twelve emotions that masquerade as anger . . ." As her voice trailed off, she began to list each of them on the giant pad, though thankfully not in that squiggly font.

1. Hurt, sadness.

A fifty-year-old guy trying hard to look thirty and wearing giant BluBlockeresque tinted glasses interrupted.

"So when I fight with my girlfriend, it's because I'm planning on breaking up with her and I'll be sad?"

"I don't know. I'd need to learn more about your relationship."

"But it might just be because I'm sad then, right?" This guy's life probably peaked in 1975 when he was a pot dealer in New Haven.

"We can discuss your situation after class, if you'd like," said Eileen diplomatically.

Suddenly I heard a rapid clicking noise to my immediate left. It was Taft giving his thumb a workout on his pen. *Clickclickclick.* He was really driving me nuts with his parade of noises so I decided it was time to take action. It was time to break out Orange Juice Carton Face. Orange Juice Carton Face was discovered in 1985 by my then roommate, Tema, after she unconscionably put an empty half-gallon cardboard orange juice container into our kitchen garbage can without crushing it so it would take up markedly less space—a handy trick I had learned from my father. Instead, because of her callous carton conduct, I was forced to reach into the garbage and pull out the hulking Tropicana container and crush it myself. The next time I saw Tema, she claims I gave her a look as if she had just intentionally burned the apartment complex down, then killed my entire family before stepping on every puppy's tail at the pound. It was the angriest look I was capable of. My eyebrows scrunched down into improbable angles, my eyes protruded from my sockets and my lips snarled as if I was about to bite someone. Welcome to Orange Juice Carton Face. Tema was petrified. It was my secret weapon and I was hoping that I could frighten Walrus Man into a clicking cease-fire with a little of my persuasive downward eyebrow movement. However,

Orange Juice Carton Face failed miserably this time. It's powerless if people aren't looking.

2. Fear, frustration.

"Anger is also a substitute for fear or frustration," said Eileen. Up went BluBlocker's hand again.

"So . . . does that mean that maybe I'm fearful of breaking up with my girlfriend and that's why I'm angry?"

The banker guy in front of me looked agitated. I wouldn't have been surprised if he stood up and told BluBlocker to shut the fuck up or he'd crush him with giant bags of money.

"Um . . . I don't know. We can discuss it after class if you'd like," repeated Eileen, who, at this rate, would never get to explain all dozen emotions.

3. Habit.

"Anger can also be a result of habit," continued Eileen. "If one of your parents was angry, then you got it!" Yep. I got it, all right. A lot of times I don't even feel that I'm the one governing my body. It's as if my mother wrote the script and I'm just acting it out.

A spindly man in the back row with all gray hair except for a small dark patch on the side (the opposite of John Henson) raised his hand.

"Is there any hope of breaking the habit?"

"Oh, sure. It just takes a lot of discipline."

Spindles seemed satisfied.

4. Reaction.

A petite lady in a sweatshirt raised her hand, but Eileen was already on to scribbling her next number, apparently trying to make up some time.

5. Disappointment based on expectations.

"This is the number one cause of anger," Eileen said with pride. "What is disappointment based on? What do you think causes disappointment?" Before anyone could respond she blurted out the answer. "Expectations. If we have no expectations, we can never be disappointed. We need to practice removing our expectations."

This was my Achilles' heel. People always seemed to disappoint me. They're late, they're inconsiderate, they're rude, they don't signal, they think they're the only person on the planet, they're unreliable. They're human. As much as I hated the way my mother treated my father, I was as guilty as she in demanding perfection. I was a drill sergeant. I was the one who wasn't human. It wasn't everybody else that was the problem, it was me. Shit.

6. Indignation in response to perceived injustice.

"Other than number five, this is probably the most common cause of anger," Eileen told us. "Indignation in response to *perceived* injustice. Remember, the injustice isn't actually there. You've just imagined it."

A large blond woman who probably had the night off from stripping interrupted.

"So if anger is imaginary and so is the injustice, why do we get angry so much?"

"Because anger is our default emotion when it should actually be set on 'happy.'"

"I'm not having a visceral connection to what you're saying," said the probable stripper, showing off her vocabulary. Maybe she was one of those strippers who *was* putting herself through school.

"We have a tendency to rehearse things in the negative," Eileen said. "How come we never choose to rehearse things in the positive? Like we never say to ourselves, 'Where am I going to find the room to store all my money?'"

The banker guy released a wry smile.

Eileen was right. My mind always raced over to the negative, not even stopping along the way to rest in the gray area. It was all part of my mother's pattern of teaching people a lesson by punishing those who wronged her. Since she was largely immobile, she relished picking up the phone and threatening legal action against insensitive doctors who had allegedly misdiagnosed or mistreated her or mail-order companies that had yet to refund her credit card for a returned purchase. And my mother would settle for a hollow victory, even if she knew the lawyer would cost her more than she'd recover. It was always the principle of the matter. It was probably also a way for her to avoid feeling helpless. Somehow I doubt that she would have wasted all this energy on trivial things if she wasn't trapped in her bedroom twenty-three hours a day.

7. Feeling out of control or victimized.

I thought about how often I considered myself a victim and would then use my anger to transform the other party into one. The collie/dogpark fiasco; the time a comedy booker in Vermont told me an anti-Semitic joke and I leaped over his desk and threatened him; the semester I sued Emerson College because the TV Performance professor gave everyone the exact same critique; the night some Nets fans at the Meadowlands refused to move their coats from empty seats which prevented my father and me from moving down from our obstructed views, resulting in me erupting at the five of them and actually assigning my dad to "deal with the guy with the red beard."

8. Needing to be right.

Before Eileen had finished crossing the *t* in *right*, BluBlocker spoke up.

"My girlfriend always needs to be right."

Eileen ignored BluBlocker's latest comment and went on to explain that one of the mental exercises she uses before employing anger is the "one-year rule."

"Will you remember the inciting incident one year from now? Chances are 99.9 percent that you won't. You won't remember a friend being twenty minutes late, you won't remember a waiter bringing you the wrong meal, and you won't remember when your morning newspaper's been stolen. And if you do, you've got quite a memory."

I liked Eileen's one-year rule.

My mother hasn't been wrong since the day she got MS. It's as if she's the '72 Miami Dolphins. Undefeated. And I can't even remember her saying the word "sorry" in a sentence. I fear that I've become just as competitive. I had to win even the most mundane and minuscule of battles. And if I didn't go for the jugular, I felt like a doormat.

"Remember that being right is the booby prize. Someone else is wrong. You're right all alone," Eileen concluded.

Nancy constantly reminds me of this when I find fault with friends. I'll whine to her about people who served us nothing but bread products for dinner or others who just talk about themselves, never asking us a single question, or that couple who canceled on us at the last minute on a Saturday night. As good as our relationship is, Nancy doesn't want us to end up old, friendless and alone. Which is always a possibility when you're married to me.

9. Displaced responsibility.

"Own your behavior," said Eileen.

The gist of this is not to blame stuff on other people or inanimate objects. If your toast is burned, don't yell at the toaster. If you park too close to a pole and scrape it when backing out, don't be angry at the pole. I agree. Be angry at the people who put the pole so close to the wall! What do they think? Everyone drives M.G.s?

10. Faulty belief system (perception).

"The other day I was driving back to my condo complex," Eileen said about an event that probably happened to her last century. "And there was a car going five miles per hour. *Five!* Right in front of me on this one-lane road where I couldn't pass her. I was angry! It took me ten extra minutes and the only reason I didn't honk and yell is because she lived in my development. Well, guess what? When she finally pulled over to her building, it turns out that she had been balancing a huge bouquet of flowers on her lap that someone had given her as a birthday present. It was her birthday! And all along I thought she was just driving slowly to annoy me."

This just made me angrier. I don't give a shit if it's *her* birthday *and* her car's birthday. Put the flowers in the backseat, in the trunk, put 'em in the passenger seat and seat-belt 'em in; I don't care what you do with your flowers but don't go one-seventh of the speed limit!!! That *is* modifiable behavior. You don't have to carry your gifts on your lap, idiot!

11. Not forgiving yourself and others.

"When you don't forgive, it's like taking poison and waiting for someone else to die."

"I think my girlfriend cheated on me, but I can't prove it," BluBlocker piped up again. I wondered how many other people were there for relationship problems. For all my ills and troubles, at least I've always had good relationships with women and kept my anger with them to a minimum—perhaps because that's the one sacred part of my life in which I won't allow things to get fucked up. It wasn't pleasant watching my parents interact. I wanted that part of their lives to skip a generation.

"If I forgive her, do you think I'll be less angry?" he continued.

"I really don't know enough about your relationship—which, *like I said*—I'd be glad to discuss with you *after* class."

Now the anger teacher was getting angry.

"Y'know," the man wearing sunglasses indoors continued, "I'm on my fourth read of *Mind Over Mood* and it *still* hasn't sunk in."

"Among other things," Eileen muttered. I half expected the class to make "Oooh" and "Ahhh" sounds like the Sweathogs when someone said something outrageous on *Welcome Back,*

Kotter. At least this was taking my mind off the adjacent man with the hyperactive pen and world's oldest piece of gum still rummaging around in his tongue house like a gym sock in an endless dryer.

12. Excuse for avoidance behavior.

Eileen scribbled the final entry on her gigantic flip pad. Underneath that little pink kitty sweater, she was seething. Her adrenal glands were releasing cortisol, epinephrine and other stress hormones; her heart rate was accelerating, blood pressure was rising and her digestive and immune systems were shutting down.

Our assignment for the week was to write down each thing we got angry at and then decide into which of the twelve categories it fit. I was hoping to have my first anger-free week so I'd have nothing to share with the class.

"I'm not going to get angry this week," I assured Nancy, who was propped up in front of the television watching *American Idol.*

"Okay."

"No, I'm serious. It's going to be my first anger-free week."

"I'm proud of you already," she said while hitting pause on the TiVo. "Can we discuss it after this is over?"

American Idol was her favorite show in the world and my least favorite thing on the planet to hear or see. Just glancing at Ryan Seacrest in my living room was making me angry. I nodded to Nancy and went upstairs.

"I'd like to know what your week was like," asked Eileen, now wearing a pink sweater with a white cat on it. As she addressed the class, she didn't even look at the side of the room where BluBlocker was sitting.

This time the class had quite a few empty chairs. I had chosen to arrive early rather than my customary really early so that I could pick somewhere that didn't have two consecutive available seats next to it. This would ensure some distance from Taft, who would probably be humming as he smashed tiny cymbals together for the next two hours. I sat one seat away from an older Russian man who was preparing to record the class with a cassette tape recorder half the size of his head.

A woman in front of me told the class that she didn't have anger issues of her own. She was only concerned with reacting to the anger of others. As Eileen explained that the anger of others is equally important to manage, I rehearsed what I would say about the week if I suddenly had the urge to share.

Two days prior, I got enraged in a supermarket. I went inside and bought one item, a prepackaged salad, and was livid when there was only one register open and nine of us wanting to exchange our money for food. Why were all the other registers closed in the middle of the day? This was bullshit! This was both number 5 (Disappointment Based on Expectations) AND number 6 (Indignation in Response to Perceived Injustice)!!! Eight-fifty for some lettuce and lettuce sauce! You'd think they'd have enough cash to hire a second cashier!!!

I removed my laminated card from my wallet while in line and selected this for perspective.

Take the "me" out of the equation; it's not "happening to me"; things are just happening.

Nonetheless, I remained angry until the automatic doors allowed my salad and me outside.

"My chemotherapy really drained me today," Eileen casually interjected, while I continued my inner rant about my salad. "Do I feel great? No. But moving on with my life is important." Jesus fuck! She had cancer! This went totally unmentioned last week. She was teaching the anger class with cancer! I knew that technically cancer wasn't contagious, but anger is and anger leads to cancer. And she knew so much about anger because she *was* angry! That was probably one of the first five ingredients in her body. I added "cancer" to the short list of things that would kill me if I didn't manage my stress better.

Then Eileen nonchalantly segued back into the anger syllabus. But my mind was stuck on her cancer.

All of a sudden the supermarket incident seemed pointless. Everything did. So what if I had to wait in line an extra five minutes? Wasn't standing around calmly for five minutes a lot better than having my body pounded by radiation week after week and throwing up a lot? And would my health insurance even cover cancer treatments?

I should be happy every minute of the day. Just being able to walk down the aisle of a supermarket should make me joyful. I was an educated white guy born to middle-class parents in America who had all the components of a healthy body and I was throwing it all away. How much easier could my life really be? What the fuck did I really have to complain about?

I looked around the room to see others' reactions to the chemo news. Nobody showed any emotion, except for a fortysomething guy on the opposite side who must've been at least 90 percent American Indian. I'm surprised there weren't more of them in the anger class. At least *they* have a right to be angry. We stole their country and practically injected whiskey into their bloodstreams and in return gave them a bunch of blackjack tables. That's fair, right?

I couldn't think about anything but cancer for the remainder of the class. I should just be thankful I could run errands. I should just shut up.

8

STRETCHING

For the next few weeks I was noticeably less agitated, sedated almost. I didn't want my fate to be a bitter guy in radiation who was given x percent chance to live. I also didn't want anyone feeling sorry for me, especially since if I did get cancer, it would only be because the tension I created in my body was like a telepathic Evite for bad cells.

But after a month, thoughts of Eileen in her pink and white cat sweaters faded, as most "I swear I'll change my life immediately if I can be assured of not getting cancer" affirmations do. I was again on the verge of threatening the next stranger who forgot to hold a door open for me with Orange Juice Carton Face. Despite the influx of added Zoloft, my brain remained a swirling mass of frantic synapses, as if my head were a pinball machine—but instead of a single ball getting flipped around off bumpers, dozens of shiny silver spheres remained bouncing about in the game known as "My Skull."

Not only were magazine deadlines stressing me out, but sitting in one position for long periods was starting to compress my spine. My joints were so tight that when I twisted my back, every vertebra cracked so loudly it sounded as if someone were shooting off fireworks in my chair.

Nancy suggested yoga.

"It'll change your life," she proclaimed.

"I'm sure it will change my life. *Anything* you do technically changes your life," I said, showering her with reason.

"C'mon, it keeps you present and loose! It's like ballet without the mirrors!"

"Ballet without mirrors? Is that supposed to make me want to go?"

"You get to wear baggy clothes . . ." Her voice drifted off.

"I've already tried yoga and I hated it."

"Bikram isn't *real* yoga."

Years ago I'd heard people discussing the magic of Bikram at a barbecue. Bikram is the first name of an egotistical litigious maniac. In his yoga routine one practices the same twenty-six poses in the same exact sequence class after class while some idiot wearing one of those hands-free microphones on his or her head sits condescendingly on top of a small wooden throne. Not only has Bikram trademarked this sequence of poses that have existed for thousands of years, but he sues anyone who attempts to replicate the sequence without a franchise fee. Oh, one more thing: the room is heated to 105 degrees. So basically, one works up a totally artificial sweat that could be acquired by sitting in a car in rush hour in August with the air-conditioning off. Bikram is a dick. And I hope he sues me. Then I'll countersue him for stealing my patented walk and ending each spoken sentence with a brief pause. I'm surprised this Bikram assfuck allows anyone to even use the temperature of 105 degrees without winding up in court.[4] I sometimes reheat my chicken at home at that exact temperature, just to annoy him.

So after one class I knew Bikram wasn't for me. But my back and I were getting desperate. As of my fortieth birthday, I estimated that I had lifted weights for a total of 13,000 hours. Here's the breakdown: between ages fifteen and thirty-one I moved barbells and dumbbells into the air six days a week for a minimum of two hours a session; between thirty-two and thirty-six, I had tapered off to four days of ninety-minute workouts; between thirty-seven and forty I was down to approximately four hours a week. So not surprisingly, for the last

---

4. In July 2006, prosecutors in Los Angeles charged Bikram with operating a yoga studio without a permit and nine other criminal counts. Bikram has threatened to move his headquarters to Honolulu. I'll drive him to the airport.

twenty years my body has been stiff and in considerable pain. Weight lifting became a convenient scapegoat for much of my hyperactive, destructive, stressful, disease-activating behavior. Hopefully a daily stretching regimen would help me escape the grip of barbells so I could stop blaming them for everything. I decided to try loosening up my body to take some of the pressure off my mind.

One Friday evening I made the pilgrimage across town with Nancy to Billy Wolf's yoga class. Since I'm an even tenser passenger than driver, I drove. The only trouble was, unlike lifting weights, where one can just show up pretty much whenever one feels like it, yoga takes place at a preordained time. Battling rush-hour traffic and a deadline, I was more coated in sweat from the drive to class than from Bikram's thermostat.

When we arrived at the top floor of an old warehouse-type building, I was shocked at the number of svelte women lying flat in the cavernous basketball-court-sized studio. It looked like a really healthy cemetery. In the back, several students were stuffing money into a large plastic box which had a hand-written sign that read "Suggested Donation: $15." So technically, I could have just dropped a paper clip in there and I wouldn't have been breaking any rules. Instead, I stuffed three tens into the slot and secured two of the handful of non-mat-occupied spaces near the middle of the room.

The class was 5 percent straight men, 15 percent gay men and 80 percent women (100 percent of whom were gorgeous). Had I been single, I would've immediately dropped all career aspirations and started studying for my yoga teaching certificate. The room began to fill up even more and the nearby mats, which were already too close to me, got even closer. I now had people no more than a pen-length away on all four sides. Despite being surrounded by beautiful women in spandex, I was still claustrophobic. Plus, I didn't know what the hell I was doing and now it would be impossible for the svelties not to notice.

Then "he" walked in and you could practically hear the gasps of delight. Billy Wolf looked like Peter Frampton if Frampton had dyed his hair black and worn a tight tank top to highlight his stupendous core strength. The women's eyes followed him as he zigzagged his way down to the front of the studio.

"That's Billy," Nancy whispered to me.

"I figured it was either him or some guy who prefers doing yoga wandering around the room instead of on a mat."

"Shhhh!"

"You're the one who started this conversation."

"Okay, let's begin!" Wolf spoke with authority in every syllable.

We started with a series of warm-ups called "sun salutations," which resembled calisthenics from gym class.

"Downward dog!" he barked.

Wolf instructed us to keep our movements slow and to hold each pose for five breaths while he pranced around the room and never demonstrated a thing—other than fifteen different ways to sneak up on attractive ladies and legally touch their asses. How did we even know he was any better than we were at yoga if we never saw him do even the simplest of poses? Maybe he was just a horny surfer with some business acumen. If he had corrected anything I was doing (which didn't happen, since I wasn't equipped with a vagina), I was planning to say, "First let's see *you* do something, Mr. Know-It-All Stretchy Guy!" But predictably, he never came anywhere near me.

"Remember," Wolf boomed, "the space *in between* breaths is what's really important." It's hard to believe that after forty-plus years on the planet, I still had to be reminded how to breathe, but, just as I'm an awful chewer, I was thankful for any advice I could get on how to use my lungs and diaphragm.

The poses evolved from the top of a push-up (plank pose) to the middle of a push-up (chataranga) to pulling and scooping your body forward at the bottom of a push-up (upward dog) and then back to turning your body into a giant V (downward dog) with your palms flat and your heels on the ground—at least in theory. I could've been wearing stilettos and the back of my heels still wouldn't have been anywhere near the floor.

I was consistently out of sync with Nancy and the rest of the class, lucky to be just one pose behind. It was usually more like two or three. As beads of sweat jumped off my body, many of them landed on nearby mats. Being the considerate yogi I was, I continuously attempted to wipe up my perspiration while simultaneously dodging the flailing legs of those in front of me, and elongated arms behind me.

My muscles didn't know what was going on. They had grown up exclusively contracting and had no idea what it felt like to stretch. Every square inch of my body was so tight I could barely get my hands past my knees on the forward bends while limber ladies around me all effortlessly put their palms flat on the ground, and a few bendy freaks, their elbows.

We then did some poses where one hand goes over a shoulder while the other one loops behind the waist and they're supposed to meet in the center of your back. Yeah, right.

"For those of you less flexible, you may need to use a towel to bridge the gap," said Wolf as he managed to inappropriately touch nineteen attractive women within the course of that sentence. Even with a beach towel I would've been unable to have my hands meet. In fact, if there were anything dangerous placed on the middle of my back, like a grenade, I'd have zero chance of reaching it. It was yet another price to pay for all my heavy lifting—I didn't even have access to half the areas on my body.

A blond girl directly to my right gave me a dirty look for what I thought was no reason. I had been continually mopping up my sweat for maximum karmic results and had no idea why I deserved her visual wrath. Until she whispered that I was breathing on her.

Another adjustment to be made. Unlike in weight lifting, where one breathes through the mouth, yoga breathing is supposed to be done exclusively through the nose, which contains tiny hairs to help filter the air. Plus, breathing through the nose, no matter how vigorous, wouldn't propel your air, and potential halitosis, onto a neighbor. I whispered "Sorry" back to blondie and employed my nostrils as I was told.

"Equaminity amongst the intensity," said Wolf.

I always thought the word was "equanimity," but maybe he knew an ancient Indian way of saying it. In any case, I didn't shout out my correction.

The purpose of holding these difficult poses for inordinate periods of time while breathing through them is to get one not to flee difficult situations. The rationale goes: if you can stay calmly balanced on one leg with both arms held in the air, then keeping a cool head when the bank messes up the address on your checks should be easy. Equanimity amongst the intensity. Or equanimity. Hey, it's his class.

Despite my limited yoga skills, this was exactly what my body needed. I was pumping blood to new areas and it felt great. From now on, no more lifting anything heavier than a blue piece of rubber I could do poses on. I would gradually reduce my free-weight intake and this would be my new, healthier addiction. I was looking forward to standing on my head and walking on my hands. Maybe I'd even show off and enter Quiznos on my palms. And I would never have to ask Nancy to scratch my back and go through that endless "a little over to the right . . . no, back toward the left . . . a little higher" sequence. I would be so fucking flexible I could drive with both of my legs behind my head and out the sunroof.

As we transitioned into one-legged poses with our upper bodies folded forward to produce a T-shape, Wolf gathered up his long curly black hair and stuck it into a ponytail. As if this was his way of saying, "Hey everyone . . . my flowing locks can produce many different looks!" He then "adjusted" a variety of swooning women into proper alignment.

"You want to twist your ribs toward the ceiling and shift your gaze to the front corner of the room. . . . Now you need to drop the shoulder blades down your back so they're not pinching each other. . . . Okay, you want to get your uterus a little closer to my dick . . ." Sorry—that last one is just me being jealous.

About an hour into class we had shifted from the one-legged T-pose to the identical position on the opposite leg. After holding the position for about five seconds, my body collapsed. I couldn't move. It felt like someone had crawled into my right hip and cut all my tendons and muscles with a hacksaw. At first I was hoping it was just a really bad cramp, but after a few minutes, when the pain didn't subside, I began to worry. Nancy glanced over and just assumed that I was tired and taking a break. And I guess I was taking a break—for another forty-five minutes until class ended.

At one point Nancy whispered to me, "Are you okay?" I was about to answer "Noooooooooooo!!!!!!" but then a redheaded sveltie shushed us.

As the class wound down to slower, more sedentary floor poses, Wolf blurted out words of inspiration which basically amounted to different ways of saying: "Take it slow and savor every moment of life but live in the here and now and keep your head free from a flurry of extraneous thoughts." To be honest, I had no interest in living in the "here and now" right then. I wanted to live in the past—an hour and a half ago before my entire lower right side was throbbing as if my leg was playing really loud music through a really tiny speaker.

The group shifted into lying meditation (shavasana) and Wolf instructed us to close our eyes and let out a sigh. I let out a shrill moan while wincing.

Five minutes later, class was officially over. A throng of gals surrounded Wolf, none of whom was there to correct his pronunciation. If there had been a Sharpie around, they probably would have asked him to sign their mats.

Nancy looked concerned, but not for the same reason I was. "Ready?"

"I don't think I can stand up or walk."

"Really?"

"Yes! I'm in pain!"

"Oh God! I am *sooo* relieved! Oh, I didn't mean it that way. It's just you seemed so distracted during class. I thought you were checking out all the other women and were having doubts about marrying me."

"Is searing hip pain one of the chapters in *He's Just Not That Into You?*"

Nancy suffers from circular thinking and, like her mother, can sometimes be a little on the nervous side. However, her mother had an excuse: she escaped from Germany as a child during the Holocaust. Nancy's defense: she used to live in Manhattan in the "model district" and had lost quite a few boyfriends to them.

"Can you get down the stairs?"

"I don't think so."

This sucked! But in retrospect it was my fault. My hip hadn't just "suddenly" collapsed. It's very rare that anything "suddenly" collapses when there are no external forces. There are always warning signs. I just chose to ignore them. First there was a twinge in my hip, followed by a little more pain in the joint in some other poses, and then the final blow. It reminded me of the many times a girlfriend would break up with me, putting me in shock. These always seemed like random out-of-the-blue occurrences, but in hindsight a plethora of incidents led to the demise of the relationship and I was an idiot for not noticing at least ten of them.

By this time the class had completely emptied out and Nancy was trying to help me down the stairs.

"Ow!"

"I'm sorry, I'm not strong enough. I'll ask Billy."

But he was already out the door having iced lattes with his bendy groupies.

"I think you're gonna have to call an ambulance."

"Shit!" Nancy said as she waved her phone in the air. "My phone doesn't work up here. Sit on the top step and I'll run outside."

The good news was that the paramedics arrived quickly. The bad news was, I was leaving my first yoga class on a gurney. My hips were strong enough to squat three times my body weight, but not powerful enough to balance me on one leg. Yeah, lifting weights had been an excellent use of my time.

As they loaded me into the back of the ambulance, Nancy was about to join me when I blurted out: "Wait! We'll get a ticket if the car's parked there overnight and then we'll have to take a cab from the hospital back here! Why don't you get the car and meet me at the hospital?"

"I hate driving your car."

"Well, you're gonna have to."

"Is the phone book in the backseat?"

Nancy's a shade under five feet two and claims that she can barely see over my Volvo's steering wheel unless she's sitting on the yellow pages. Which, frankly, I have a hard time believing. She's a mere three inches shorter than the Denver Nuggets' Earl Boykins and I bet he can drive an Escalade without even sitting on a napkin.

At the hospital, they took some X-rays and an MRI and it appeared that I had torn a muscle in my hip, although the doctors didn't sound all that confident in their diagnosis. They stuttered and stammered through their conclusions as they held the film up to the lit background.

For the first time since I tore up my back squatting six years earlier, exercising was out of the question. I could barely walk and couldn't even get my shoes on without Nancy. Once in a while, if I was particularly grouchy, she would pretend to leave the house without helping me with my Pumas. I was beginning to understand how my mother felt. When you're reliant on another person and semi-helpless, little things become big things and big things become all-encompassing.

I knew the only hope of regaining my independence anytime soon was physical therapy. I was already a PT vet. After an ill-

advised fistfight during my senior year of high school outside
Mr. America's Gym in an icy parking lot, the left side of my
lower body was temporarily partially paralyzed. I wound up
going to the same physical therapist as my mother (occasionally
our sessions even overlapped) for a trio of three-hour sessions
every week, as well as doing prescribed exercises at home on a
daily basis. My diligence enabled me to avoid a back operation.

I'd also had physical therapy to rehabilitate a knee I had torn
up in 1998. I'd purchased a pair of special sneakers with giant
waffle-like pads affixed to the ball of each foot. The heel of each
sneaker was suspended several inches off the ground and the purpose of the footwear was to build up your calves so you could
"jump higher." (In hindsight, when you've over thirty, unless
you're in the NBA or Sergei Bubka, there's really no reason to
"jump higher.") Hours after my magic shoes arrived in the mail,
I went to a local park to do the specialized exercises on the in-
structional video that accompanied my new high-heeled sneakers.
I bolted across the outfield of a softball field doing drills: running
sideways and crisscrossing my legs for a couple hundred yards,
followed by a series of wind sprints. In under an hour, I tore my
knee ligaments and had to crawl to my car. The shoes didn't help
me jump higher, but they did help me not jump at all.

But this time my hip was so messed up (I believe that's the
medical term) that my attempts at rehabilitation were pointless. I went to a nearby physical therapy center and even the
simplest of tasks like riding a recumbent bike on the lowest
setting proved too painful. I was sent home. They couldn't do
anything until I regained some strength. Despite the excruciat-
ing discomfort, I can't say I was totally miserable. The pleasure
of the impending healing process outweighed the pain.

As month after month drifted by and my hip wasn't getting
any better, I needed to search elsewhere. I asked everyone I
knew if they could recommend *anyone* who might help me.

My friend Stephanie referred me to her acupuncturist. I was
totally open to the whole "sticking needles into your body"

process. Hell, I was open to anything. But ten sessions, three hundred tiny needles and $1,200 later, my hip still felt like that of an unhealthy eighty-year-old. I came to the conclusion that the entire premise behind acupuncture is that when they pull all the needles out of your body you instantly feel much better because you no longer have needles in your body. It was time to move on to the next thing. A friend of a friend of Josh's came through with a name and a number.

I walked into a tall glass building covered with tinted windows and looked for suite 301. The Pain Foundation. I was expecting to enter the waiting room to a series of people moaning. "Ohhhh, we're in soooo much pain!!!! Ohhhhh!!!!" Part of me was wondering if there were any doctors there or just a series of dominatrices who would whip the shit out of you. I was somewhat disappointed when it looked just like the hundreds of other doctors' offices I had frequented.

My appointment was with Dr. Keith Pevsner, the Pain Management Specialist. Dr. Pevsner was a jolly, energetic man resembling Mr. Carlin from the original *Bob Newhart Show.*

He looked at the X-rays and asked, "Have you ever had a cortisone shot in your spine?"

Hmmm . . . I actually had to think a minute for the answer. "I don't think so."

"Now, this *is* somewhat experimental, and your insurance won't cover it, but it probably won't hurt you . . ."

"Probably?"

"Well, you never know," said the pain guy with a chuckle. Oh, he was a hoot.

I may be a hyper-chondriac but I'm no coward, so I agreed to the injection. But I did consider what the consequences would be if (a) the doctor had a mild case of Parkinson's and his hand slipped while injecting my spine or (b) an earthquake struck just as the metal met my vertebra. Still, I happily allowed a stranger to stick a needle the size of my spine into my spine, and it hurt like a motherfucker.

"Now, call me in a week and we'll see if it did anything," said the guy holding the giant needle.

"Oh, it definitely did something."

When I got home, my hip was killing me; I could barely walk, barely sleep and I was in agony while driving. Plus, on top of everything, my spine was tender.

A week later, I was back on a table at the Pain Foundation.

"I'm sorry that the shot in the spine didn't work. I thought that the origins of your hip pain might be in your vertebrae. Would you like to try some cortisone injected directly into your hip?"

He sounded so casual, as if he were my waiter reading off the lunch specials.

"Sure, why not?"

Again, this procedure wasn't covered by my insurance, but I really wanted to go on a nice hike again at some point before I was dead. This time the needle appeared to be the length of two stickball bats taped together. I turned away as Dr. Pevsner plunged what seemed like the entire thing into my bad hip.

"Jesus Christ!"

"Let's see if this does anything for you. Call me in a few days."

A week later, there was no change in my hip. But there was a change in my bank account. All these tests and treatments were getting expensive. The shots alone were close to $1,000 apiece and Blue Cross wouldn't cover anything, so this was all out-of-pocket. These insurance companies really hold all the cards. When you're "unhealthy" you don't really have the luxury of shopping around for care and it seems only a narrow range of treatments are covered anyway. And when you're "healthy" you don't really think about insurance that much.

I returned to the painful confines of the Pain Foundation for a third time.

"Any relief?"

"Nope."

"Okay, let's try some of this." Dr. Pevsner removed a pen from his pocket, scribbled something on a pad and handed it to me.

It was a prescription for Celebrex.

"Now, be careful with these. Make sure to take them with food."

I was supposed to take 400 mg worth of these white pills with yellow stripes every day. But even with a full meal, I could feel the pills quarreling with my insides. Each one felt as if it were ripping out my stomach lining. I thought it might be my imagination until I read on the Celebrex website that ". . . stomach problems such as bleeding can occur without warning and may cause death." Of all the things that could kill me, I never thought it would be a yoga class.

Weighing a pill's potential side effects versus its healing effects can be tricky; the pain and inflammation in my stomach began to rival that in my hip. Would I need another pill to temper my stomach pain? Eventually, I'd have to take twenty different tablets every morning until I arrived at a side effect that was manageable.

Just taking a single pill got confusing at times, but juggling two seemed at least five times as difficult. Often I'd think I'd taken my 100 mg of Zoloft only to wonder whether that was actually yesterday, or if it was today but my Celebrex and not my Zoloft. I considered employing Nancy's sophisticated straightening-iron technique to help. Seconds after she leaves the house in the morning, I seem to always get a phone call.

"Did I unplug the straightening iron?"

"You always unplug the straightening iron."

"Can you check, please?"

I always do and it always is. I asked Nancy what she does when I'm not home to confirm matters. She told me that in those instances she says "I'm unplugging the straightening iron" aloud to double the chances of remembering whether she did as she's driving away. It's only a matter of time before I'm yelling "I'm taking my Zoloft!" loud enough for the neighbors to hear.

A week after I started Celebrex and five months after my yoga mishap my hip began to feel a little better. My physical therapist referred me to hydrotherapy, since water offered less resistance than land-based exercise and was easier on the joints. The only trouble was, like my father, I couldn't swim. Yes, I've tried on numerous occasions. And no, you wouldn't be able to teach me, either. But thanks. During the summers, I'd stayed after camp to work one-on-one with a variety of lifeguard-like instructors without any success. Every girlfriend I've ever had thinks she can teach me to swim. Or at least float. They're all wrong. On our honeymoon, Nancy stuck her hand under my stomach in the three-feet portion of the pool, told me to relax, then released me as I hit bottom like an anchor.

Maybe drowning would solve my hip problem.

For six months I wore a life jacket and clutched a tomb-shaped piece of Styrofoam as I kicked my way across the width of the pool. My hydrotherapist, a curvy thirty-five-year-old named Tara, often had multiple clients at the same time, none of whom was under seventy-five. They often asked me what I was doing there.

"I mean, you look so healthy," a wrinkled old woman (who was probably slightly less wrinkled when not in the water for long stretches) said. "What did you do to yourself?"

"I hurt my hip."

"How, sweetie?"

"In yoga class."

"Isn't yoga supposed to be good for you?"

"Yes."

"I broke my hip thirty years ago and it hasn't been the same. Then once osteoporosis set in, *everything* hurt."

"My shoulder's been throbbing since Korea," said an older gentleman. "And my prostate is killing me!"

"I have prostate problems, too!" I said, way too excited and loud for a large empty space with a lot of tiles.

"Aren't you a little young for prostate troubles?"

"Yep."

By the way, you'll know if you have prostatitis when your penis stops working. It's pretty scary. Imagine that one of those "Back at ___ o'clock" signs that antique shop owners leave on their doors has been hung on your groin—except there are no hands on the clock. Because even when you squeeze your glutes together, you CANNOT FEEL YOUR PENIS! Fortunately, the treatment is saw palmetto capsules, warm baths and frequent masturbation to keep the prostate busy.

"I only have one kidney," said another older woman proudly, having bullied her way into our conversation.

I realized I had more in common with octogenarians than anyone my age.

After drying off and changing, I'd head upstairs where a team of land-based therapists manipulated and stretched my limbs on a giant table in hopes of strengthening my hip. It felt as if they were playing tug-of-war with my torso. Then it was off to the recumbent bike for some more hip strengthening and light resistance exercises.

Unfortunately, as my hip got stronger so did my dependence on Celebrex. I was at the mercy of the nonsteroidal anti-inflammatory drug and, as with my Zoloft, was frightened at the prospect of running out, or needing a refill on a bank holiday. I was told by members of my land therapy team to drop down to 200 mg. However, halving the dose seemed to double the pain and set me back weeks on my PT schedule. I secretly went back up to 400 mg to go with my 100 mg of Zoloft. I really didn't need to become addicted to *two* pills, but I was equally frightened of tapering off. I even Googled "Celebrex Anonymous" to see if there was a support group. Nope.

Finally, my Celebrex habit took care of itself. I had so much inflammation from the onslaught of pills that my stomach was hemorrhaging. The ulcer diagnosed by my gastroenterologist made for an easy decision. My PT sessions were a lot more painful without pills but it was better than "... stomach problems such as bleeding can occur without warning and may cause death." And bleeding to death in an indoor pool would really freak out my new old people friends.

A scant fourteen months after being introduced to the magic of yoga, I was finally able to walk without pain. And despite having Blue Cross and Blue Shield, by the time the smoke cleared and I had paid my deductible, my acupuncturist, my team of physical therapists and the pain specialist, that one yoga class had cost me over $6,300. Yes, I had parlayed a $15 donation into a 42,000 percent loss. And that doesn't include replacing the yoga mat I'd borrowed from Nancy's friend and forgot at the studio during the gurney hullabaloo.

Maybe it was a sign to focus more on my mind.

9

SCANNING

I stood awkwardly in the courtyard of the Kabbalah Centre in Los Angeles waiting for my watch to say eight-thirty. If anyone had ever bet me that I would pay $270 to sit in a classroom listening to Kabbalah lectures for ten weeks, I would have wagered my entire checking account. Which wasn't very much after the hip episode, but that's not really the point.

Due to my yoga accident I wasn't able to exercise much, so I had some extra time on my hands and thought maybe a little spirituality would calm me down. I had heard about Kabbalah from the likes of Madonna, Ashton and Demi, but it was my friend Renata who actually encouraged me to go. Earlier in the year, she had been in a bit of a rut and needed some divine inspiration to get a better job and quit smoking. So Renata enrolled in Kabbalah Level One and moments after completing the course got a better job and stopped smoking—which the cynic in me thought could've also been accomplished through Monster.com and the patch.

I tried to convince Nancy to come. She's much more impressionable than I am, anyway. Whenever the alarm clock, VCR or microwave has all three numbers the same (1:11, 2:22, etc.), she orders me to stare at it with her and make a silent wish. My wish is always the same: "I wish Nancy would stop making me stare at things for one-minute increments."

"Come to Kabbalah with me," I begged. "C'mon! I went to yoga with you."

"Nah. But if you bring me home one of those cute red string bracelets, I'll buy you sushi tonight."

○ ○ ○

I had mentioned to Renata that I had issues with organized religion. She assured me that Kabbalah wasn't that organized. Ever since my rabbi converted to Episcopalianism, I'd been unable to set foot in *any* house of worship because of acute panic attacks. The trauma was manageable when I was a teen because my religious exposure had ended abruptly after Setzman shunned Judaism.

But when I was a freshman in college, the issues resurfaced. A group of girls in my dorm were going to High Holy Days at a local synagogue. Since they were really cute and I was really horny, it was a no-brainer to tag along. Ten minutes into the services, my head was spinning, my stomach churning, the pews swirling and I nearly blacked out. After I staggered into the bathroom and lay on the cold tiled floor to recover, it took all my strength to return my yarmulke and grab a cab back to the dorm.

As I got older, things only got worse. Regardless of the religious affiliation, freaking out, turning ghost-white and blacking out became the norm. Whenever I got invitations to weddings or bar mitzvahs, I'd either lurk in the back of the temple/church/mosque/Scientology Center so I could take frequent breaks or skip the ceremony completely and just go to the reception, blaming my tardiness on car trouble or MapQuest.

In the spring of 1999, due to a flurry of friends getting married and a desire to rid myself of this religion affliction, I called around to several doctors, described my problem and asked if they knew of anyone who could treat me. After dozens of phone calls and months of detective work, I had struck neurological-therapeutic gold. Peggy Townsend specialized in religious issues and was eager to meet me.

Ms. Townsend was a twice-divorced, wavy silver-haired Texan. She was raised a Southern Baptist, but her first husband was Catholic and her second Jewish. Despite being in her early seventies, Peggy had a quiet intensity about her, as if underneath the sheen of authority, she was a fiery gal who still got in bar fights.

"So when you go into *any* religious venue, you have these attacks?" she said with remnants of her southern twang.

"Yep."

"Are they more acute in a temple than a church?"

"No. Same."

"Do you think this has to do with your rabbi becoming an Episcopalian minister?"

"That probably has something to do with it, yeah."

"So you feel betrayed?"

"Sure."

"And is there anything specific, that you can tell, that triggers these attacks?"

"Nope. It's more of a time thing than a content thing. I can last up to ten minutes if I completely block out everything and think about sports or a movie I just saw. But if I just sit there and listen and absorb everything, I'd say I last an average of three to five minutes."

I told Peggy how religious worship makes me feel on the verge of collapse and blindness, as if God is turning me into a helpless marionette. Congregants then approach me and tell me I look deathly ill and I have to lie and say that I think I have food poisoning. My only salvation is to stumble out of the church or temple pew and lie on the bathroom floor, where I can continue to breathe deeply out of earshot of the minister or rabbi until the color returns to my skin, the strength to my legs and the sight to my eyes.

"Then what happens?"

"I slowly recover and stagger to the foyer and wait until the ceremony is over. I don't want to take any attention away from the bride and groom. And I really don't want to make a scene twice."

"Why do you think you feel like God's marionette?"

"I guess if I knew I wouldn't be here."

Peggy then slid her entire set of lips over to the left side of her face, lost deep in thought as I whirred on.

"Religion feels like a combination of begging and nagging to me. I mean, do I want to worship a God who needs me to constantly tell Him how great He is? Would the Creator of the Universe be *that* insecure? And if I'm continually asking Him for things and promising to be good in return, isn't that a little like extortion?"

Peggy's lips then quickly moved, trombone-like, completely onto the right side of her face.

"Maybe I just feel that my family's devotion to God really hasn't paid off. It all seems so futile. I don't know. Maybe He's punishing me. He punished my mom and my brother Andrew and my grandparents."

"Do you think you're an atheist?"

"No. That's the weird thing. I do believe in God. My head is just all messed up. Like I say that I don't believe in an afterlife, but on the other hand I refuse to check the 'organ donor' box on my driver's license."

"So you're agnostic?"

She was just going down a list of questions in her head now, and not listening. I had just told her nine seconds ago that I believed in a God, though not necessarily One that demanded a lot of back-and-forth chitchat.

"No. And I don't feel that everything fits so neatly into one of our preconceived categories."

Religion itself was full of contradictions. If everybody's prayers were hypothetically answered, there'd be a lot of them canceling each other out. So what would be the determining factor in who gets what? Is it based on need? Who asked first? Or is it just completely random like everything else in the universe? Even before my panic attacks started, I had always felt a little awkward about the whole sitting-in-the-same-place-and-saying-the-same-thing-to-the-same-entity-at-the-same-time thing.

"Let's get back to your panic attacks for a moment. After your rabbi left, these feelings became heightened?"

"Yes."

I didn't even tell her about the Star of David sternum grinding.

∘ ∘ ∘

Despite my occasional bouts of exasperation, I saw Peggy Townsend weekly for nearly three years, mostly talking in circles about religion to get to the root of my troubles. The answer always came back to what she had uncovered within the first seven minutes of our very first meeting. Betrayal. I felt betrayed by God that my rabbi left the temple and converted and I had felt uncomfortable dealing with Him ever since. It was as if a girlfriend and I had had a messy breakup but then kept running into each other at the hostess stand at Bennigan's.

It took two years of sessions before I told Peggy that when I was fifteen my temple was razed and retirement homes were built on the exact spot where we used to worship God. I guess I had blocked all that out.

Although discovering the origin of my problem was good information, it didn't cure me. It just enabled me to tough it out at weddings and bar mitzvahs for slightly longer periods of time before the attack swarmed my body. Even 100 mg of Zoloft couldn't fend off the meltdowns. I was barely able to make it through my own wedding. Had it not been for the 50 mg and Nancy alternating between squeezing my hand so hard it changed colors and burrowing her fingernails deep into my palm to distract me, I probably would have passed out. And, had that happened, she probably would've smashed the entire cake into my face and then run off in her giant white shoes.

So perhaps now you can understand why paying $270 to stare at a group of Hebrew letters at a Kabbalah Centre for two and a half months seemed like the last thing I'd ever do. But Renata had been a chain-smoker with limited professional skills, so I decided to give it a try.

The Kabbalah Centre was inside a stone building that looked to be a hundred years old, which in Los Angeles is the equivalent of the ancient pyramids. (Incidentally, I'd prefer to spell "Centre" as "Center"—however the former is the way it's spelled on the black hardcover Kabbalah 101 binder that they gave me.)

I had forty minutes to kill before my first class, so I browsed around in the adjacent Kabbalah gift shop. It gave me pride that these pseudo Jews were into marketing their cult, or whatever it was. I firmly believe that's why Christianity really took off and Judaism didn't. Marketing. Think about it—they have a guy's face (and often his body) on necklaces, posters, stained-glass windows, sculptures, air fresheners and bumper stickers. We have a six-pointed star—which can easily be confused with the Houston Astros' logo. Quite frankly, it's amazing that there are any Jews up against a PR blitz like that. We'd be much better off having a guy's head on our jewelry, like Ed Asner or Michael Landon.

There was an eerie sense of peace inside. All of the customers/students/already-brainwashed humanoids had portions of smiles glommed onto their faces and fashionable red strings on their wrists. The cashier, who looked like Lisa Loeb had she opted for the tinted tortoise-rimmed glasses, turned to me.

"Excuse me? Can I help you find anything?"

I wanted to blurt out: "Yes! My SOUL!!!"

Instead I just doled out the standard "No, thanks."

The courtyard connected to the gift shop had four or five round black metal tables with matching folding chairs. Since everyone seemed to be shopping, I was able to snag a chair next to a tall potted plant that kept swatting me in the face whenever a breeze approached. As I became irritated and started swatting it back, a flood of people came streaming into the courtyard. The early classes had finally let out and I could find my classroom and grab a seat—in the back near the doorway in case the material became too "religiousy" and I had to flee for the bathroom floor.

As I barged into the classroom to secure a suitable seat, other students trickled in behind me. The "fiftyish housewives whose kids have finally gone off to college and who now have way too much time on their hands" contingent; the "English is my second language but I'm a goddamn knowledge sponge, so give me what you got and I'll absorb it" gaggle; the "hot girls who might be fun to fuck but are obviously nuts" faction; the "horny guys who just want to meet someone—anyone!—and are tired of singles' bars and online dating" group; and the blond Jew who is trying desperately not to have an anxiety attack by not making eye contact with the scattered Hebrew letters on the walls.

I sat next to an attractive red-haired girl who was most likely an actress. She seemed so emotionally fragile, as if all of her tears were lined up and ready to leap out of her eyes at a moment's notice. I wondered if this was a cumulative effect from life or if she had just had a fight with her boyfriend an hour ago. I grew tired of waiting for class to begin, so I introduced myself, making sure she saw my wedding band and throwing in the term "my wife" about ten times within the first minute so she wouldn't think I was hitting on her. Her name was Heather and as I glanced down at her bag on the ground, I saw one of her headshots poking out of the top. I was right. Actress.

"Are you okay?" I asked.

"If I was okay would I be here?" she snapped back, a tear trying valiantly to escape from her eye. "Are *you* okay?"

"I guess not."

The instructor entered. Whether he had a closely cropped beard or an awesome five o'clock shadow I wasn't sure. A dark blue suit covered his slight frame and he wore a yarmulke that blended in quite nicely with his hair color, which thankfully made it harder for me to notice. (Yarmulkes make me queasy, too.) The only reason I even knew he was wearing one was the occasional glint off the silver clip that affixed it to his scalp. He walked to the podium in the center of the room and spoke into the microphone, which I thought was totally unnecessary for such a small group, but I later learned was used to record the session so that anyone who missed a class could pick it up on cassette during the week.

"Hello, everyone," he said in a British accent.

He'd better be British. Impersonations annoy me.

"My name is Ethan and I'll be instructing you for the next ten weeks." Good. His accent was consistent; he really was British. Ethan seemed to be about my age and possessed a natural charm that went with his warm face and bright smile.

"First thing we're going to do is go around the room and tell everyone the reason you're here."

A bald man wearing too much cologne was first.

"I want to achieve financial success."

Then why not take the $270 you just spent and put it into a mutual fund? was my instant internal response.

"Well, you *will* achieve financial success if you open your mind and heart to Kabbalah," Ethan assured him. The bald man looked elated and probably would've dabbed on more cologne in celebration had he not already finished the bottle.

"I'm having trouble meeting men since my husband and I separated," said a chunky housewife.

"You will resolve *all* your relationship issues with Kabbalah."

Or with a diet and not wearing polka dots.

And so we went around the room with everyone explaining why they were there and Ethan promising them that this was the perfect solution to their problems. Issues seemed to involve either relationships or money. Except for Heather, who just wanted "to become a better person" and nearly cried by the time she had reached the third word in her sentence.

Finally it was my turn.

"I'd like to control my anger so I stop inflicting disease on myself."

Although I knew that the second half of my statement opened a can of worms and would provoke at least one additional question from Ethan, I didn't want to mention just the "controlling my anger" part. I didn't want anyone thinking I was a wife-beater or thug.

"Your anger inflicts disease on yourself?" Ethan asked.

"Yes. I need to be calmer. You'll just have to trust me on that."

"Well, you will resolve all of your health issues with Kabbalah."

He smiled and then consulted his notes hidden behind the podium and explained that *Kabbalah* in Hebrew means "to receive."

Everyone in the class eagerly jotted that down.

"Did you know that according to medical science, we utilize only four percent of our brain capacity?"

Heather looked depressed about that information.

"And, according to science, we still fail to perceive ninety-nine percent of our universe."

Uh, can I get some footnotes and sources here, please? Exactly "who" in science has proclaimed this? It's like those bottles of special shampoo that say "Dermatologist Recommended." So technically, one dermatologist on the planet could have said, "Yeah, I'd use that instead of battery acid on your itchy scalp."

Ethan continued: "*Our* world is called the one percent. It is a world of chaos. It's like the Murphy's Law planet, basically. Whatever can go wrong, will go wrong. However, the realm beyond is known as the ninety-nine percent. The purpose of Kabbalah is to bring the ninety-nine percent and the one percent together."

Okay, I get it. We're not privy to everything that's going on. I was pleased that there didn't appear to be too much deep religious mumbo jumbo. I wasn't in the mood for an attack right now.

"We are all disconnected from our souls," announced Ethan as if he were telling us the price of a plum. "The only way to reconnect is to understand the concept of the Light and the Vessel."

Basically, once upon a time, each of our souls was part of one infinite soul—the Vessel. The essence of this Vessel is a desire to receive. A cup is a Vessel, while the coffee that goes inside is the Light. So, the bigger the Vessel, the more you'll attract Light, energy and success. It all seemed to make sense.

Ethan explained that the main objective of Kabbalah is to

transform your nature from Reactive to Proactive. The Light is Proactive, the Vessel is Reactive. Kabbalah teaches you to embrace the difficult situations of your life by focusing on your reaction to these obstacles and not the external circumstances.

I was certainly Reactive and not Proactive. It was just hard to ignore other people most of the time. I would love to employ the turn-the-other-cheek strategy instead of my eye-for-an-eye mantra. However, my affliction contains a huge incongruity: that people are oblivious of me yet these same strangers are specifically saying "fuck you" to my existence. Which is the same behavior that my siblings and I constantly criticize my mother for.

Due to the multiple sclerosis, my mother has been unable to move around and has understandably gotten heavier. She also fell and broke her hip, had it replaced and had her thyroid removed, altering her metabolism for the worse—all before the age of fifty. Thus, on the rare occasions that we went out to eat, she would feel as though everyone in the restaurant was "staring at the heavy cripple." At the same time, she would be insulted that these same people inside the eatery didn't notice her when she was creeping along the aisles with her two canes and one husband. So, wait a second . . . everyone at his or her respective table is simultaneously talking about you *and* doesn't know you exist . . . huh?

"By shutting down your Reactive System and letting in the Light, you can dismantle every obstacle in life," Ethan went on. "However, it's not as easy as it sounds. Because there is an opponent in this game and his name is SATAN!"

Uh-oh.

Not surprisingly, Satan has a game plan, too. While we're trying to become Proactive, Satan is trying to make us Reactive. (FYI, in the handouts he's also referred to once as "Stan," perhaps to either throw us off track or make us Proactive to sloppy spelling.) While we should be trying to share the Light, that rapscallion wants us to hog all the Light for ourselves. I bet Satan spends a lot of time here in Hollywood.

"The whole purpose of Satan is to challenge us," Ethan told everyone. "He does this by dispensing momentary pleasures that will soon plunge us into darkness. Satan loooves to dangle instant gratification in front of our noses."

Another drop of water emerged from Heather's tear duct.

"But we *can* defeat Satan! Does anyone know how?"

I wanted to yell out, "Poisonous cupcakes!"

One of the housewives' hands shot up.

"By giving him the cold shoulder?"

"Uh . . . what's 'the cold shoulder'? I'm quite sorry, but we don't use that expression in Britain."

"It means ignoring him."

"Ah, yes. No. Kind of, actually." Ethan was easily flustered if he had to stray from his script. "The key to defeating Satan is to shut down the Reactive system and remain Proactive at all times."

I proceeded to write "Ignore Satan" in my notebook.

For the next week, I tried to shut down my Reactive side and stay Proactive. Although putting all my focus into *not* over-reacting should take markedly *less* energy than exploding, in reality it seemed to require even more force. When a guy at a diner blatantly cut in front of me at the cashier, I shut down my Reactive side and let him. When I saw my neighbor not clean up after his dog, I remained silent and said nothing. When a woman in a pickup truck nearly crashed into me in a parking lot because she was looking down at her cell phone while simultaneously backing up, I merely smiled at her over-size vehicle and let her selfish behavior roll off my back, conscious of my reaction and unconscious of her action. Then the following morning I stepped in my neighbor's dog's shit and wanted to strangle him. Still, my life was improving in tiny steps. I would definitely go back to Kabbalah.

At the beginning of the following class, one of the hot crazy chicks raised her hand.

"Yes. You have a question?" asked Ethan brightly.

"Is it true that the Kabbalah water has healing powers?"

The question was delivered in such a monotone staccato, it sounded like a rehearsed question for an infomercial. This girl had never shown any interest in anything Ethan had said and all of a sudden she was asking a question as if she were on an audition. I looked around the room to see if she was reading a cue card off to the side. The girl had definitely been asked to ask this, probably while meandering around the gift shop—which is where Ethan hung out before class.

"The Kabbalah water *absolutely* has special healing powers." Remarkably, Ethan was even worse at acting than the woman who asked the question. "There have been tests done on it throughout the world that prove it can change your body's properties. Believe me, this water can change your life."

I remember that Nancy said she tried the water once at a party and that it rejuvenated her. On the other hand, she doesn't drink enough fluids and is always dehydrated, so whenever she drinks anything she's grateful.

"What's in it?" asked the balding cologned guy unexpectedly.

"We can't divulge the special formula but suffice it to say that the molecules have been altered to produce really special results."

How can you alter the properties of water? I wasn't much of a science guy, but isn't it simply H_2O? I mean, what the fuck have these Kabbalists done—tossed in an extra molecule of hydrogen for good luck? Despite my skepticism, all of the Kabbalah water was sold out within ten minutes after class. Part of me was disappointed.

"If you hit a home run in baseball"—I could already tell from the change in his cadence that Ethan didn't know shit about sports; he was just giving the analogy he was required to—"you'd be pretty happy, wouldn't you?"

The class nodded like a group of bobblehead dolls.

"But if you later learned that the only reason you had hit that home runner"—home runner?—"was because your father had arranged it with all the other fathers before the game . . . how would that make you feel?"

The class looked none too pleased.

"Exactly!" chirped Ethan in an accent that was really starting to get on my nerves. "It wouldn't mean a thing because you would have had your bread without earning it. That is called the 'Bread of Shame.'"

Everyone's hands wrote down "Bread of Shame" like good little students.

"Removing the Bread of Shame is one of the greatest gifts that the Light has given us. Every obstacle we face is a bar of gold!"

There was some overlap from my Anger Seminar. I guess if we always got what we wanted, the world would be a pretty boring, unsatisfying place. Plus, I'd rather my dad not stick his nose into my Little League games so I knew I was solely responsible for my lowly .231 batting average.

This Bread of Shame seemed sensible. I went to college with a guy named Darren whose parents were filthy rich. Darren never had to worry about money or what he wanted to do with his life. Throughout college, while I was working the night shift in a liquor store or being a concierge at a snobby condominium complex, I was always a little jealous of Darren's situation. Twenty years later, thanks to the world of compound interest, he's even richer but hasn't accomplished anything and is drowning in his sea of free time. Darren is miserable.

Before our fifth class, I accidentally spilled my complimentary piping hot tea all over my groin area. Fuck! "Bread of Shame, Bread of Shame!" I repeated to myself. Yep, these third-degree burns on my inner thigh were like a bar of gold that would teach me to slow down and not try to walk and sip at the same time.

Ethan walked in and confidently slapped his notes down on the podium.

"All of our various destinies are all already scripted—just like a movie."

The pens started scribbling.

One of the housewives raised her hand.

"So we have no control over our destinies?"

"Well, yes and no. You see, we can choose the movie that we'd like to be in, but the movies themselves are already done."

"Can't we recast?" pleaded Heather.

"No. All of the movies are completed and predetermined."

I heard the cologned bald guy mutter "That sucks!" to himself.

"But although all of the movies are already done, there is one bit of good news." Ethan tried to cheer us up. "There are many, many movie theaters. The universe is like a giant multiplex and we have the power to choose whichever movie we'd like!"

A collective sigh of relief emanated from everyone's mouth.

"So we CAN rewrite the movie, then?" Heather declared hopefully.

"No," repeated Ethan. "We can walk into a different theater, but we have no control over the story."

"So if we switch movies, then doesn't that change the casting and the story line of the new movie that we're entering?" one of the perplexed housewives asked.

Ethan looked puzzled. I guess he hadn't been in Hollywood that long.

"Not exactly," he said, repeating his stock response to ward off confusion. "Most people never change movies. But those who *do,* have the power to alter their destinies!" Ethan's voice nervously proceeded to rise three octaves. "You see, if a coworker is bugging you, you simply switch movies and your nemesis stays in the old movie."

"But what if he follows you into the new movie?" I wanted to ask, but didn't.

"Most people never change movies," continued Ethan. "Remember that all possible destinies exist in these movies, which are all found in a parallel universe."

Suddenly, I hunched over as if I were about to throw up.

"Are you all right?" Ethan asked.

"Yes. Just a torn cornea from Boston. I'll be okay."

Ethan moved on as I furiously rubbed my eyelid to stimulate moisture. If Heather ever tore her cornea, she'd be in great shape.

Ethan went on to tell us that energy manifests itself as twenty-two forces, which just so happen to be the twenty-two letters of the Hebrew alphabet. Coincidence? Hmmm . . . Because of their shape, sound frequencies and vibrations, these twenty-two Hebrew letters act as antennae that connect us to these energy forces. The example given to us was this: if you hit a musical triangle with a stick, then place another triangle near the first one, the second triangle will begin to vibrate as well, thanks to the "transference of energy."

Out of the corner of my eye, I actually saw Heather write down the words "Buy pair of triangles."

"Through the power of the Hebrew letters, we can alter our DNA!" announced Ethan, as if he were suddenly a scientist.

Alter our DNA?

The class nodded in synchronized awe.

Okay, now I was getting a little fed up with this fictitious bullshit. How could you just blatantly lie and tell a roomful of adults that staring at some letters can change the internal building blocks of your body? Since I'm not well versed in science, I asked my pharmacist to triple-check and he laughed, before adding, "It's impossible to change your DNA. You're stuck with it."

I was seething over the DNA propaganda for the next week. It was irresponsible, ignorant and blatantly false. Even more disheartening was that no one in the classroom, including me, challenged the "fact."

At the beginning of our next class we were given a laminated sheet of paper with the seventy-two names of God in the form of six dozen different sequences of Hebrew letters that were supposed to connect us to powerful, positive energy sources in the universe. I hadn't read Hebrew since I was thirteen and had no idea what any of this collection of letters meant. Plus, they usually made me feel faint.

"It doesn't matter," Ethan assured us. "All you need to do is scan them."

The letters were arranged in an eight-by-nine grid. I still had no idea what he was talking about.

"Right to left, one day, then try up and down another time."

Heather's hand went up, extra dramatically.

"So all we have to do is make eye contact with each one of them? Is that what you're saying?"

"Exactly. You'll be rewarded. Good energy and good things will happen in your lives if you do."

As I rolled my eyes, Heather noticed the look of scorn on my face and turned to me and whispered, "Sometimes you just need to take a leap of faith."

For the next two weeks, every night before I went to bed and every morning when I woke up, I spent a few minutes scanning the letters and words that I could neither read nor pronounce. There was certainly no harm in this scanning and it actually soothed me. I was scanning the shit out of those letters. Thankfully, Nancy was understanding. She was happy it quieted me down. Had she mocked me in any way, I had the "Staring at the Clock at 4:44 and Making a Wish Nonsense" ready to throw back in her face.

I started to think that maybe Heather was right. Maybe part of the healing process requires some suspension of logical thought. Maybe a leap of faith is the only way to get over a hurdle. For the first time in my life, I decided not to worry about logic. Logic was more likely to make one crazy than calm. Believing in this stuff wasn't so hard, after all. It was suspending my disbelief that was the tough part.

"The Zohar is an amazing, amazing book. Or rather, set of books," Ethan told us proudly at the beginning of our next session.

The Zohar was a set of twenty-three giant encyclopedia-size

hardcover volumes that would monopolize a bookcase. They were entirely in Hebrew and you weren't expected to read them, just to scan the pages. He went on to tell us of the magical powers of a set of Zohars that were mailed to Iran in the 1980s against the Iranian government's wishes. The government then tried to ship the books back to America but SOMEHOW the Zohars wound up returning to the same Iranian warehouse—as if the "To" and "From" labels had been reversed. A few months later, the entire warehouse at the airport burned down—EXCEPT for the area where the Zohars were being stored. (Perhaps they're flame-retardant?) Then a few months after the fire, a major earthquake struck Iran and the fault line mysteriously split very close to where the Zohars were being stored and allegedly millions of Iranian lives were spared.

And the stories went on. A woman who had breast cancer scanned the Zohar and her tumor disappeared. A man whose son had disappeared a decade ago scanned the Zohar and the son turned up at his doorstep a week later. A thirty-two-year-old Kinko's cashier who was making minimum wage scanned the Zohar and was still making minimum wage. Sorry, but there's no reason to roll your eyes at someone who's trying to improve himself.

The Zohar, all twenty-three volumes, was conveniently available in the gift shop for a mere $415. Nearly two dozen books that I couldn't read and wouldn't understand—for LESS THAN $500!? Instead of getting angry about the expensive books with the outlandish claims, I let my Proactive mind downgrade my cynicism of Ethan's sales pitch to that lone internal quip, then slid my laminated sheet with the seventy-two names of God out from the middle of my notebook and scanned them.

10

SITTING (STILL)

I spent several minutes each night scanning the Hebrew letters and several hours each day listening to Ethan's classes on cassette as I drove around Los Angeles. I was starting to feel better and, most important, hadn't contracted any illness or had so much as a cold since I began my quest for calm. I decided to pursue the spiritual angle further.

I had always been impressed with Buddhists. I admired them for never knocking on your door to push their Buddhist propaganda on you. And you wouldn't see a Buddhist preaching the virtues of being Buddhist on street corners. And Buddhists didn't have missionaries who traveled to foreign countries to brainwash the general populace into renouncing their non-Buddhisty beliefs. Plus there were no fundamentalist Buddhists. Buddhists were unflappable, calm and relaxed.

So maybe that's why I didn't hang up when Tim, a guy I exchanged numbers with at Kabbalah 101, called me to brag about the Buddhist temple he'd attended. He told me to check its website for "some cool shit that was comin' up" and I did, periodically, but nothing really appealed to me. There was a Special Statue Filling Day in which one stuffs holy objects into various Buddhas for offerings to the spiritual guide, Puja. But that just seemed like busywork. I also wasn't interested in The Bodhisattva Vow—a five-week class that was "a practical guide to helping others." This was all about me right now. Then one full-mooned night, surfing for salvation, I hit the mother lode: the Weekend Sitting Seminar. Sitting still = being still. Being still = not being high-strung and overly aggressive and subsequently getting ill. Count me in, Buddhists! I just hoped it wasn't too late to sign up.

"Where are you going?"

"Buddhist temple to sit still. Wanna come?" I asked Nancy.

"No, thanks. All I do all day is sit."

Nancy had just started a new job writing on a sitcom in which she sat around a large conference table with thirteen other writers pitching jokes and story ideas all day. I didn't think she'd be interested in sitting in less comfortable chairs on her days off.

I made the fifteen-minute pilgrimage to a gritty neighborhood near Dodger Stadium. Parking was pretty easy, so I was already in a jubilant mood when I arrived at the temple, which blended in with the rest of the adjacent boxy concrete architecture, as if it were a public library or a bank. I admired the anonymity of the structure.

Naturally, I was a half hour early. Despite my overzealous punctuality, I was surprised to see two dozen other soon-to-be sitting-stillers already milling about, all cradling cups of tea, near a large rectangular table. The assortment of people ranged from flabby sixty-year-old men wearing flannel to skinny thirty-year-old men wearing flannel to forty-five-year-old women wearing baggy flannel-blend yoga pants who looked like they hadn't had sex since 1997. The three things everyone had in common were a ponytail, no makeup and the appearance of being stoned. Oh, and flannel.

Before I could get my own cup of tea, I was greeted with a large bear hug that caught me completely off guard. First of all, I'm not a big fan of the male hugging thing. Even a high five is too much guy-on-guy affection for my taste. Second, if you absolutely *do* need to touch me, don't hurt me in the process unless I've done something wrong, in which case be blatant and just punch me in the stomach or break a beer bottle over my head. The hug monster was Tim from Kabbalah.

And Tim is one large man. All you really need to know is he's six feet seven and used to be a bodyguard for Van Halen. Despite being five feet ten, whenever I hung around Tim I felt like he could've carried me around in a Baby Björn.

"Look at this! Ya made it!" Tim announced as he slapped me on the back a little too hard.

We walked over to the registration table and I learned that the seminar was $50 for one day and $80 for the entire weekend. Tim was signing up for both days and I thought that was my best value as well. Besides, I wasn't there for the *Saturday Sitting Still Seminar*. I wanted the optimum results and one full day of remaining motionless on my ass surely wouldn't suffice. I handed my check to the woman on the other side of the table, and she pointed us inside.

The place was packed with about two hundred sitting-stillers crowded around an empty oversize wooden chair that stood in the center of a red velvety pulpit that also housed a large six-foot statue of Buddha. Apparently there were more people than I had imagined with nothing better to do than a weekend of nothingness. At least *I* had an excuse. My Zoloft would soon be useless. What were their rationales? And why couldn't they simply stay at home and sit still if they were this ardent?

There were three choices of places to sit. On a pillow on the ground near the front. No, thank you. Sitting on the ground in any form would make me extra cranky. That's why picnics were always out of the question unless someone could guarantee that there would be a table involved. I'm also one of the few people on the planet who are not fond of hammocks. I'm always afraid the slightest of moves will flip me off that drooping piece of canvas as if the hammock knew judo.

My remaining choices were chairs with a pillow on them in the middle of the temple or in the back on a cold metal folding chair. My glutes voted for the former, as did Tim until he spotted some moderately attractive women in the back. Anyway, when you're six feet seven you really shouldn't be up front unless you're in a particularly spiteful mood, in which case you might as well go for it and wear a top hat, too.

So Tim and I split up, which was fine because I'm happily married and not trying to get laid and you can't talk during this thing anyway. Before he ventured off to hit on some blonde in the back, he gave me another unnecessary bear hug, nearly breaking my floating rib.

I sat down on a cushiony chair between a grossly overweight thirtysomething guy with a salt-and-pepper beard and a twentysomething woman who looked a little like Debra Winger. I considered my options briefly and started chatting with Debra.

"So, why are *you* doing this?" I asked.

"Because I just got back from three weeks of silence in Laos and I need to get back into my meditation."

"Wait. You were silent for three entire weeks?"

"Yeah. It was awesome."

My mother had once gone three weeks without speaking to anyone in the family, but that was because she was pissed at us. My mom is the best grudge-holder on the planet. She'll undoubtedly hold another one against me for this paragraph.

I was amazed that a human being would voluntarily not utter a word for nearly a month *and* commute 12,000 miles to do so.

"What was so awesome about it?" I asked.

"It totally reconnected me to who I am."

"Yeah, but what did you do for the three weeks?"

"Meditate."

"But, I mean, how did you eat? You must have had to say something to somebody. A 'thank you,' a 'please.'" I was getting on her nerves even before I employed logic.

"Do you ever meditate?" Debra asked.

"I've tried but I can't anymore."

"Why not?"

"Because I've ruined it for myself."

"You can't *ruin* meditation." I felt as if I was certainly accomplishing that for the people seated near us who were trying to get a head start on the proceedings.

"Well, I did. When I was living in England I was in a punk band[5] and I tried to meditate to a tape with this Austrian guy speaking but then the bass player sampled his voice as the lone vocals for a song and now meditating makes me even more hyper."

"You need to just listen to gongs," she advised, and shut her eyes and put her fingers in that circular position as if she were making the A-OK sign. But she wasn't. Because she hated me. I should have chatted up fat beardy instead.

Seconds later, at ten o'clock on the dot, the female monk—who could have starred in the Sinéad O'Connor biopic—emerged from a doorway at the side of the pulpit and welcomed us to the event. She didn't speak for very long, which was fine with me because her voice was so soft it sounded like the world's shyest child's—possibly explaining the popularity of the cushions on the floor up front. However, I *was* able to hear that our lunch break would be at twelve-thirty, which I was hoping we didn't have to sit still for. There would probably be healthy food, too—rice cakes, lentils and chamomile tea. I suddenly realized I was glad I was doing this. Monk-y girl then sat down in the giant wooden chair and closed her eyes. Our two days of nothingness were under way. Hooray.

As I shut my lids and drifted off into alleged stillness, I could only think of one thing: how fucking boring this was already. I was among a bunch of freaks—men with no muscle tone, women who were cute but looked angst-ridden and asexual old people in dashikis. I should've stayed out until five in the morning drinking. Then at least I could've appeared to be spiritually superior by sleeping through the day. But no, I had to get nine hours of sleep because I wanted to be fully rested.

---

5. In 1996 I formed a band in London called Invasion of Privacy. We intended to set up our equipment in random places (which we never got around to) in hopes of getting arrested (which they never got around to).

This had suckiness written all over it. And I had one of the cushiony chairs. Plus, it's not like you can look at the person next to you and cheat, either.

When you're trying to meditate and any thoughts drift into your head—regardless of what they are—you're just supposed to ignore them. In general, I'm not a very good ignorer. Instead I just repeatedly compile lists of things I want to do that day, that week, that life. List after list after list. I was hoping to just shake my head and erase them all like an Etch-a-Sketch, but whenever I did, new lists would form. I sneaked a look at my watch, hoping that lunchtime was approaching. Technically it was approaching, but unfortunately extremely slowly as it was only 10:06. Talk about a long weekend. How do those Buckingham Palace guards do it? To me there's no worse job on the planet. I couldn't do that job in sweatpants lying down.

I could have been at the Dodgers game with my buddy Jeff. Box seats! Roy Oswalt pitching! I immediately dragged my mind back to positive thoughts and reiterated how important this seminar was. Once I broke through a wall or two, the rewards would be great, probably. Patience. Patience. Relax. Breathe. Patience. Listen to your breath. Okay . . . that's enough for now. Peek at your watch . . . go ahead . . . peek! It's gotta be close to noon by now. Go ahead and open your eyes . . . Shit! 10:09! How did the Dalai Lama stay still? Maybe he was just really lazy.

I thought about how I'd always equated sitting still with some sort of punishment. Like if you did something bad in grade school, the teacher would make you go and sit in the corner. Or if you committed a crime, you were expected to sit motionless in the back of the police car. When exactly did sitting still evolve into a positive thing? It stank to high heaven. If Amnesty International found out that the U.S. government was simply making the Guantánamo suspects do what I was doing right this moment, it would constitute torture. I decided right then I would never speak to Tim again.

My mind raced through all the things I'd rather be doing at that moment. Picking up trash on the side of the highway in the dead of winter in Nova Scotia seemed like a fine option. So did ironing some dress shirts. I'd even rather have been making subs at a deli. "Sorry, we're out of Cheddar. Would you like some goat cheese on your honey-baked ham, sir?" (I know, most delis don't have goat cheese, but mine would be a *special* deli.) Suddenly, nothing in the world seemed tedious. Except what I was currently doing.

I didn't know how I would survive another seven hours and fifty-one minutes of this today, let alone another full day tomorrow. In fact, fuck tomorrow. Tomorrow was out. Maybe by giving myself a reward of somethingness the following day I could make it through this day of nothingness.

I wondered what Debra was thinking about right now. This must have been child's play for her. I absolutely abhor cell phones and only use one in an emergency but I wished some thoughtless drone's Nokia would go off. And if it did, I was hoping that the ring tone would be a really annoying song like "Bad Day" or Beethoven's Fifth. I'd even have settled for a LeAnn Rimes tune. More nothingness.

Eighty bucks for this bullshit. Now I wished they had accepted charge cards so I could have disputed the charges, or at least bitched on the phone to the American Express customer service rep. What a waste of time and money. For eighty bucks I could have probably bought one of those robot vacuum cleaners. I'm not even sure what they cost, but I know that the price has come down considerably, kind of like when calculators were around $300 in the mid-'70s. Personally, it would take a lot less energy for me to do my own vacuuming than worrying that the little dish-shaped robot was bouncing into my coffee table and chipping its rosewood legs. Are people that lethargic that they can't even push their own vacuums anymore? I'm sure it's only a matter of time before there's a robotic shaver that darts horizontally across your face while you're sleeping. You'd just have to remember to tape up your eyebrows, of course.

I sneakily opened my eyes. Everyone in the room looked really at peace in a culty sort of way. Tim and Debra both had giant smiles plastered on their faces to accompany their nirvana. I was in hell. 10:17. Okay . . . Enough of this crap. I had to get out of there. And this time I meant it. Enjoy your vortex of nothingness, Debra Winger doppelgänger and flabby facial-haired dudes! Adios, Tim! I'll be listening to the traffic report in about six minutes.

I rationalized that my departure would be a good test for the other sitting-stillers to see if a fellow stiller's exit would distract them from their task. I was actually doing them a favor. C'mon, let's see just how good all you people are at not moving. I stood up, and as I eased my way past several other participants in this sadistic experiment, no one's body language changed an iota—even though the aisles were so narrow I either nudged them with my knee or stepped on their feet (all accidentally; I'm not that big an asshole) as I made my way toward the doors. No one in the entire temple even flinched; no one raced up from the non-cushioned chairs to seize my superior cushiony seat; no one followed me out. I thought that maybe my quitting would be an icebreaker and that I'd be the Pied Piper of movement and be joined by at least a dozen others who would exclaim "Wait up! We're going with you! This blows!" But I left alone.

I looked at my watch in the hallway. 10:19. Nineteen minutes out of sixteen hours. I'd lasted a mere 2 percent of the curriculum. I'd like to think I was 2 percent calmer, but I was probably 25 percent less calm than when I initially sat down. This whole fiasco was aggravating. I was beginning to appreciate the no-nonsense Zoloft.

I figured I might as well use the bathroom before I began the grueling four-mile drive home. Maybe I would sit still on the toilet lid for another minute and bring my grand total up to an even twenty. My search for the john brought me back into the kitchen, where I saw a large bowl sitting at eye level on the counter. I approached it in hopes that there would be some berries or yogurt-covered pretzels or carob-coated macadamia nuts, but instead it was filled with personal checks. Apparently Buddhists believe in reincarnation but not safes. Now, most of me wanted to skip the bathroom, contract my bladder until I got home and just leave right then. But some of me wanted to see if my $80 check just happened to be in that thing.

I riffled through the bowl and found the check I had made out about a half hour ago. Wait a second. What was I doing? Why was I holding my check in my hand? I couldn't possibly take it back. That would be wrong, and very un-Buddhisty. But on the other hand, $80 was an awful lot of money to pay to sit down for less than twenty minutes. That's over $2 a minute per ass cheek. About the only expense the temple would incur would be the wear-and-tear of the seat cushion, but that would be negligible. God, this was so wrong. I felt like I was in an episode of *Laverne & Shirley* and I was both Lenny *and* Squiggy. I looked around to see if anyone else was nearby. Of course not. Everyone was next door pretending to be paralyzed. This was too easy. Basically I was stealing money from a room full of paraplegics. But it was *my* money. But it still wasn't right. But on the other hand, neither is charging someone eighty bucks to sit still. Especially someone who couldn't sit still. They were preying on the weak—me! I could have probably called the Better Business Bureau. Why did I think this whole thing would be a good idea? I could never sit still. I hadn't been able to sit still for forty years—why would today be any different?

I picked up the check, stuffed it into my pocket and darted off into the bright sunshine. I was back in my natural habitat, moving around frantically. And, as weird as this sounds, it felt good. But I knew it shouldn't have.

11

WALKING & STANDING

A work friend of Nancy's was over and they were having wine on our patio when suddenly I heard someone honking really loud. It was a neighbor two doors away in our tiny cul-de-sac. I'm not going to lie to you. It can be really frustrating living in a tiny cul-de-sac. Parking here is a hassle. Although we have a three-car driveway, there are only a pair of public tandem spots available for the other four houses that share the cul. So there's usually *some* honking going on, just not the impolite, forty-five-second beeps that were happening now.

Beep! Beeeeeeeeeeepppp!!!! Honk! Hoooooooonnnnnnnnnkk-kkkk!

I yelled out the window. "Shut up, motherfucker!" (Sorry, Zoloft.) I raced out and saw that another neighbor had blocked him in which, like I said, happens a lot with tandem parking in a cul-de-sac. The neighbor and I exchanged words, and it was not a good exchange rate for him that day. I asked him to be a little more considerate of waking the other neighbor's toddlers, as my voice cut right through the trees and echoed throughout the canyon, waking toddlers in distant neighborhoods.

When her friend left, Nancy was furious.

"Why did you have to scream out the window?"

"Sorry. I forgot you had a friend over."

"Even if I *didn't* have a friend over, you shouldn't yell at the neighbors. You shouldn't yell at anything. Unless a coyote wanders into our yard. *Then* you can yell!"

"Okay. Please stop yelling."

It's not like I wasn't trying. After the Buddhist debacle I

went back to scanning Hebrew letters and realized that they did have a calming effect. So I enrolled in Kabbalah 102. But before the new charges had even appeared on my Visa, I discovered that Kabbalah has just enough information for the initial course. Each class was redundant and Ethan seemed to speak even more slowly, repeating things over and over and over again, belaboring points and trying to drum up audience participation, hoping no one would notice the lack of actual content. It was impossible not to notice. Although I still scanned occasionally, I was through with any organized Kabbalah. And its special water tastes like Arrowhead. My time would be better spent with my laminated anger card.

Early the next morning, Nancy and I heard some rustling in our yard. We assumed it was a squirrel or raccoon scampering through our leaves. When we left for our respective days—she to make money, me to have a mandatory dermatologist checkup for my Zoloft—we noticed something different about our yard. A big human shit was sitting in our driveway. Yes, it was big, it was human, and it was definitely shit. And no, it wasn't a dog's shit. We know all the animals that live on our block because some of the people don't clean up after them. By necessity, Nancy and I have become skilled at identifying what shit belongs to what dog so we can inform the respective owners. Copper is the largest of the bunch and she weighs fifty-five. This was definitely the shit of a 200-pound human. Nancy freaked out.

"Someone shit in our driveway!"

"I know! Who do you think it was?"

"Hmmmm . . . just a guess but maybe the honking guy you were yelling at yesterday."

"Oh."

"You have *got* to stop yelling at the neighbors!"

"I know."

"Then stop! Now when we're gone he's going to vandalize our house and we'll be *wishing* he was shitting in our shrubs!"

I'd never seen Nancy angrier. Including the time the Town Car driver insisted on carrying her laptop and then left it in the airport parking lot.

We collected the shit in a large Tupperware container for evidence and Nancy went over to the perpetrator's house to question him, like a *CSI* detective. I would've gladly gone but I also would've gladly pissed on his plasma and force-fed his own shit to him. He opened the door and let her in. She paced in his kitchen, tossing out threats.

"We have your shit, and therefore your DNA and we're calling the police[6] . . . so if this was you, beware! They'll be questioning you!" She waved her little fist in his face.

Nancy returned, satisfied with her confrontation, and reported his denials to me in my car, where I'd been sitting and seething. I didn't feel well. My arms and legs trembled and my colon began to palpitate. My visit to Dr. Tamm couldn't have been better timed.

"How are you feeling?" he said with sternness, as if it were a demand and not a question. "You seem really tense."

"I thought I was getting a little calmer, but then a neighbor went to the bathroom in our driveway."

"Have you been lifting weights?"

"No. I hurt my hip in yoga and it's been over a year now since I've lifted."

"Good."

During my new non-lifting era, my body had loosened up considerably and I didn't feel like a robot when I walked. Now I could no longer blame my hypertense life on dumbbells. The entire weight room was officially acquitted.

But my mind and body still weren't working together.

"I don't really want to up your Zoloft again but you're still so tense I think it's necessary," announced the doctor of skin.

---

6. Nancy later called the police and was informed that unless we saw the guy shitting or had witnesses, we didn't have a case.

"Then I'm up to 150 mg?"

"Yes."

So instead of reducing my intake another 50 mg, I was now just one step away from the maximum dose. My experiment in calming down was moving in the wrong direction. I felt like a loser.

Dr. Tamm reached into his wallet and pulled out a business card and handed it to me.

"I also want you to see this guy."

I stared at the card.

"Have you ever taken Tai Chi before?"

"No."

"Go. I think it'll help you."

The Tai Chi instructor that Dr. Tamm recommended happened to be ninety-two years old. Although I didn't know what the point of Tai Chi was, I was intrigued enough to drive forty-five minutes each way just to see a really really old guy who still had a job.

I'd taken Tae Kwon Do for several years in my twenties, but that pretty much consisted of dressing in white and kicking things. It also made me even more paranoid. As a bodybuilder, I just assumed that only people bigger than me were dangerous. With Tae Kwon Do, it became apparent that anybody could potentially beat the living shit out of me. Which stressed me out even more, even while I was kicking things.

Hopefully Tai Chi wouldn't have the same effect.

I pulled up at eight-twenty in the morning in a sweatshirt and sweatpants to a 1930s house in a dingy suburb of Pasadena and looked for hints of where the Tai Chi'ing would be taking place. I wondered if I was at the right house number but on the wrong street. But I was too anal for that. Then I noticed an Open sign hanging at the top of the driveway. As I headed toward the only clue I had, I saw an elderly Chinese man with a gray Fu Manchu mustache and a decent head of hair seated behind mounds of paperwork at a small desk in the front of his open garage. He definitely needed to buy some filing cabinets. One gust of wind could have obliterated nine decades of records.

"Mr. Chow?" I said with trepidation. I wanted to make sure I showed the proper respect and didn't seem like an American tourist in Paris in the late 1970s with loud Bermuda shorts and a camera slung around my neck, hollering about the lack of hamburger joints.

"Dr. Tamm recommended that I see you."

"Come in," he solemnly answered in a bassy voice that sounded like an Asian James Earl Jones. This guy certainly didn't look ninety-two. More like sixty-two. Maybe he was lying up to get more business.

"You have to buy shoes."

I already had shoes but apparently not the officially licensed and approved Tai Chi footwear. I followed him into the back of his office slash large garage slash shoe store, where I paid twelve bucks for a pair of black fitted slippers that looked like my little sister's ballet shoes.

"How much are classes?"

"No classes here. Just shoe store," Mr. Chow said with a straight face before a hint of a smirk slid out.

I was easily persuaded to sign up for two classes a week, which set me back sixty-five bucks a month.

I put on my slippers and Mr. Chow led me back into the largest chunk of what used to be his two-car garage. Only instead of a couple of Jettas, there were a handful of older potbellied men with long hair and mustaches wearing sweatpants and T-shirts moving very . . . very . . . slowly. It was as if they were all auditioning to be one of those guys on a street corner who paints his entire body silver and pretends he's a robot so strangers will drop a dollar in his robot tip jar. But even slower than that, actually.

I went to a vacant spot in the dojo—aka the giant garage—and almost slipped and fell. The floor was made of some kind of slate, but it was really shiny and polished: the equivalent of walking onto a frozen pond in Capezios. Apparently this is the way the floor's supposed to be because everyone else there seemed to be pretty upright and stable. I checked the bottom of my slippers to see if I had forgotten to remove a piece of cellophane or something, but I hadn't.

I'd expected some sort of organized class, where Mr. Chow would stand up front and teach us all the same things, like the Anger Seminar, yoga and Kabbalah, but this was more of a free-for-all where each man just did his thing and ignored everyone else. Mr. Chow would then walk around and correct everyone individually. But I didn't have anything to correct yet. At least I thought I didn't.

"The root of your tension is your posture," he announced to me with the utmost confidence. And a little too loud, frankly.

"My posture?"

"Yes. You have too much curvature in your lower spine. You need to stand up more erect."

So maybe all of my aggression and illness could have simply been solved by not slouching?

"Like this?" I asked as I made my body stiffer than a West Point cadet and nearly toppled over onto the shiny surface.

"No! You need to drop your chest, you need to pull your shoulders forward and you need to shoot your hips up."

I did as I was told but felt like a Picasso painting. Mr. Chow just shook his head. This posture criticism was all very surprising to me as I had always been under the impression that my body was *too* upright. But I wasn't going to argue with a ninety-two-year-old guy who would probably outlive me.

"Let's see you walk now."

I walked gingerly across the garage but before I had taken five steps was getting yelled at again. This guy was all business. And not only would he easily have won the gold medal in the Senior Citizen Glare Olympics, but I just noticed that two of the four walls were covered with gigantic swords, which I'm sure weren't being used to cut vegetables. I had better be ultra-polite so he wouldn't dice me up.

"You don't walk properly."

Wow was I a fuckup. And damn was this floor slippery.

"You need to relax," he said with ninety-two years of frustration.

"I know." Why do you think I just handed you seventy-seven bucks ten minutes ago?

"Also your breathing is all wrong."

"I'm breathing wrong?" I asked incredulously. I didn't know how to walk, stand or breathe. It was a miracle I was even alive.

"You need to breathe through your upper back and not your lungs."

I just smiled and did as I was told. I wasn't going to get defensive or answer his statements with questions anymore.

Finally it was time to learn the "form." I had to memorize a series of movements that Mr. Chow performed alongside me, nearly all of which I found very confusing. He barked out sequences like "paint the walls with your fingertips," "carry the ball," "single whip," "thread the needle," "shut the window" and "eat the cowboy's hat." Yeah, I made that last one up. But it was still very confusing.

In slow motion I had to raise my arms above my head, then slowly bring them down as if my fingertips were painting the wall in front of me while I simultaneously bent my knees as if I were hovering over a couch. Then I'd shift all of my weight onto my bent left leg and then lift my right foot and place it perpendicular to my body. Then I'd pretend to carry a large beach ball from the left side of my body to my right. You get the idea. I did a bunch of really slow movements, which collectively must've taken about ninety seconds, and then had to repeat them again and again and again on my own, until class ended. I also integrated a few original movements, like turning my head toward the clock—in slow motion, of course—to tabulate how many more times I'd have to do this before I could do things at normal speed and not be afraid of falling.

As I "painted the wall" and "carried the ball" I watched the other students engrossed in their own movements. There was one older guy who was great at moving slowly—except that he kept taking a break to drink out of a giant thermos every five minutes and then would dart to the bathroom the opposite of very slowly every eight or nine minutes. I think the overweight bearded guy next to me had Parkinson's, because his entire body never stopped quivering for the duration of the class. Which simultaneously saddened me and frightened me; I often had quivery hands. Only one other person in the class was under fifty—some shaggy-haired guy named Steve who was a veritable pun factory.

"Hey, Mr. Chow. Did you read today's newspaper?"

"Not yet."

"Well, corduroy pillows are really making *headlines*!"

Then Mr. Chow would laugh as if it was the funniest joke he had heard since Chiang Kai-shek moved his government to Taiwan and Parkinson's guy would shake even more radically.

"Hey"—Steve was going for an encore—"good news. You don't have to lock your doors anymore."

"Why not?"

"Because the Energizer Bunny was finally arrested. He was charged with battery."

More laughter and quivering. Hadn't Mr. Chow spent one hour of his ninety-two years flipping through a *Mad* magazine?

The hour was finally up and I was relieved. I felt I'd wasted more time and money on yet another shenanigan. Even the slippers were a horrible investment. Plus, to be honest with you, I'd rather see a medley of really bad impressions than hear a single pun. However, oddly enough, the rest of the day I was noticeably calmer and happier. It was a miracle.

I guess the monotony made my brain realize that I didn't have to be busy all the time. By focusing on the minutiae of the poses, the breathing, the shifting of my weight and the standing, I didn't have room for other nonrelevant thoughts to drift into my head. I had unlocked the secret to Tai Chi in a single class! I felt recharged, but not in a hyper way like when I wake up after a good night's sleep. Maybe this Mr. Chow guy was onto something. I'd devote my life to Tai Chi, practice in the mornings, play chess at night and live a long, long time with my perfect posture and flawless breathing.

I practiced each morning at home, then went back to class a few days later. Mr. Chow gave me several new movements and corrected the ones he had already given me. Apparently, I wasn't very good at "carrying the ball." Then he asked me what I did for a living.

"I'm a writer."

"Oh, writer. Let me see how you write. Sit down."

I followed him to a wooden bench attached to the wall and sat.

"Now type," he commanded.

This was the weirdest writing sample I had ever been asked to produce. I halfheartedly pretended to type and for some reason would occasionally smack an imaginary return bar as if I were using a 1923 Underwood, perhaps to make him feel more at home.

"Uh . . . should I be typing anything in particular?"

"No, just type."

"Okay." I kept flailing my fingers in the air. Then I heard a long sigh.

"You're not a good writer."

My fingers stopped. Fuck you, I thought. Which I believe he sensed.

"I mean your posture is awful for writing," he qualified. "Just a second."

Mr. Chow disappeared into his cluttered office and returned carrying a tissue box.

"Put this on your head."

"Huh?"

"Put this on your head."

Once again, I did as I was told.

"*Now* type!" he said.

I couldn't even see the imaginary paper I was writing on anymore. Although the upside was that if I sneezed I wouldn't have to look for tissues. I'd be wearing them as a hat.

"So I'm supposed to write with a box of tissues on my head?"

"Yes. It will keep your head and spine in line and help you to relax."

"You sure?"

"Of course I'm sure. You need to do as I say. I've been teaching this method for almost seventy years."

"What if it's a box of doughnuts instead?"

"No doughnuts. Tissues."

I wasn't as funny as Steve.

Once again, this stupid shit seemed to work. Even while I was driving, my seated posture was much more erect and I was especially relaxed. And I didn't have neck and shoulder pain when I was at the keyboard for long stretches. Give me more, old man!

As I entered the dojo for my next class, Mr. Chow shook his head in disgust.

"*Still* not walking properly."

"What now?"

"When you walk, you need to rotate each of your thighs clockwise while each shoulder rotates counterclockwise."

"Thighs clockwise . . ." I felt totally bowlegged. If I were in the presence of a cowboy, he'd think I was mocking him.

"Shoulders counterclockwise."

"Shoulders counterclockwise."

"And your pelvic area tilts forward and up. Toward the sky."

"Pelvic up and forward."

"Forward and up."

"Isn't that the same thing as up and forward?"

"No."

"Okay. Forward and up."

Mr. Chow then slithered behind me and gave me the Heimlich maneuver and I nearly discharged my banana bran muffin on his slippery gray floor.

"Did you think I was choking? What was that for?"

"You need to have your stomach lift your chest. You can do this yourself by making a fist and shoving it into your belly. Go ahead. Try."

I followed instructions.

"You just made yourself two inches taller," he declared. "How do you feel?"

"Taller . . ." I said rather weakly. Although it felt as if I had lacerated my spleen from punching myself in order to acquire the extra height. But I actually *did* seem taller. I was a giant!

I proudly walked around the dojo with my newfound height, just to see if I could remain taller while in motion.

"No!"

What did Mr. Chow want now?

"Yes?" I answered in my new taller voice.

"Don't swing your arms. The ball joints in your shoulders don't move. Only the arm from the elbow down moves. Just your forearms."

"Got it. No arm swinging, just forearm swinging."

I practiced walking around my house and giving myself the Heimlich. Nancy told me it looked like I had a stick up my ass, but if it stopped me from making neighbors defecate in our yard, she was all for it. I became obsessed with scrutinizing a profile of my hips and lower spine in the full-length mirror in our bedroom. "Forward and up . . . counterclockwise . . . clock-wise . . . no ball joints . . . shoulder blades go toward opposite walls like wings . . ."

At parties, I became more concerned with how perfect I could make my posture than to whom I was talking. More often than not, people asked if there was something wrong with me. "Were you in a car accident?" I told them my Tai Chi teacher had instructed me that this was the way to live a better life, and I was interested in a better life and stop judging me and where the hell was the cold beer but not that weak Bud-weiser crap and maybe they should stop slouching or the rest of their existence would be miserable. I became a connoisseur of posture, correcting my friends' aloud and strangers' inside my head.

Though apparently I wasn't doing a very good job with myself. At the next class, after studying me as I entered the dojo, Mr. Chow told me my brain was in trouble.

"God! Now what?" This was maddening.

"You're walking with your brain."

"Well, isn't it hard to walk without it?"

"You need to put all the emphasis in your feet. Only then will you walk properly."

"I thought I *was* using my feet."

"Too much brain. Not enough feet."

Was this guy fucking with me?

I was told I had to "demote my brain from five-star general to three-star general and put one star in each foot." Mr. Chow wanted me to step and push down with each foot and then use the bottom of the foot to pull the body forward so the stress from the spine would be reduced. Christ! Concentrating on the minutiae of breathing, standing, walking and typing was now making me *more* tense and, even worse, draining my Zoloft reserves. Fortunately, Steve's voice was about to take my mind off myself.

"Hey, Mr. Chow . . . do you know of a good massage place?"

"Sorry, I don't."

"Darn. Because I fired my masseuse yesterday. She just rubbed me the wrong way!"

Shut up, shaggy! You're not five!

The next time I went to class, there was a sign over Mr. Chow's garage door that said Closed. Closed? Why was it closed? Was there a Zamboni cleaning the dojo? Did the wind flip the sign and no one had bothered to flip it back? Had he fallen in the shower? Unless he'd died, I was pissed. I'd just wasted forty-five minutes driving there and now the ride home in rush hour would be even longer. Bread of Shame! Bread of Shame! Just like Kabbalah Ethan said, "Every obstacle we face is a bar of gold!"

I got my answer as to Mr. Chow's whereabouts when I bumped into punster Steve and running tiny-bladdered man in the dojo's driveway. Steve told me that Mr. Chow was an actor and probably had another audition that he'd forgotten to tell his students about. He had just tried out for an Olive Garden commercial and had allegedly recently finished shooting a Citibank spot with Ellen DeGeneres. I learned that this guy with the gray Fu Manchu mustache who was born *before* World War I was getting more acting work than Antonio Sabato Jr. *And* he had an agent!!! *And* a manager!!! I wondered if Mr. Chow nagged Ellen DeGeneres on the set of the Citibank commercial to sit up straight and push her pelvis forward and up . . . or up and forward . . . Y'know what? I don't really care what he says, they're the same damn thing!!! I knew Steve was angry too, because no puns left his mouth over the next sixty seconds.

"This actually happens a lot," Steve told me.

"It does?"

"Yeah, it used to really annoy me when I lived farther away."

"It's not right," chimed in tiny-bladdered man, spilling some of his thermos juice on his Dockers.

"I can't even believe it," said Steve. "I mean the guy's ninety-two and he's a working actor. I'm thirty-two and I can't even get an audition." Steve was bitter and had a dark side, which I found much more palatable than incessant wordplay.

"It's not right!" said the guy clutching a thermos. "He should at least call or e-mail us."

"He's gotta tell us some other way besides leaving a sign on his garage," pleaded Steve.

"It's not right," repeated tiny-bladdered man. "It's not right."

Ten seconds later, Parkinson's guy showed up, spotted the Closed sign and just slowly shook his head, which was already shaking.

The four of us decided to confront Mr. Chow at our next class. This behavior was unacceptable, regardless of how old he was. Besides, using his age as an excuse wouldn't work; the guy was still driving across town on his own, walking unaided and upright and memorizing lines. Surely he was capable of remembering to tell his students about schedule changes.

On the other hand, he was just eight years away from living an entire century. Maybe the elderly deserve more slack. Maybe we should all just let this go. Besides, angering an old guy with a lot of giant swords on his walls probably wasn't the best idea in the world. But it was never too late to learn manners and gas was really expensive. Something needed to be said.

Even though I was the newest Tai Chi'er, they wanted me to be the one to confront Mr. Chow. Steve had been going to him for nine years and had never said it bugged him, so it would be weird if he piped up now. And tiny-bladdered guy seemed to have enough of his own problems.

"Mr. Chow . . ." I stammered before our next class. I was about to give a ninety-two-year-old man a lecture about responsibility. "Your students, um, we . . . would love it if you could . . . y'know . . . next time you're not able to teach class . . . for *whatever reason* . . . if you could notify us . . . somehow."

"You have my phone number on a scrap of paper somewhere," trembled Parkinson's.

Mr. Chow looked embarrassed.

"Lots of students to call," he said. "I don't always have time."

"Well, you could get a website." I wasn't being an asshole. He was computer savvy. He had a G3; I saw it buried under papers in the garage. "That way all you'd have to do is literally post one announcement on the Internet and people could check it right before they left for class."

"Website?" Mr. Chow looked intrigued or like he was going to fight me. "Okay. I'll get a website."

Both sides seemed satisfied with the outcome, and a couple of weeks later Mr. Chow's website was up and running. I read on it that he was starring in a video game in Seattle and would be gone for four days the third week of the next month. Cool. The system was working.

A week later I was practicing "carrying the ball" and "grasping the swallow's tail" when Mr. Chow said he had an announcement: he was raising his prices for the first time in six years.

"Why?" Steve looked devastated. He was struggling to make his payments as it was.

"To help pay for the web designer and website upkeep," Mr. Chow answered before shooting me a look of disdain.

Despite the wave of animosity, I continue to go back to the dojo to do my assortment of slow-motion poses. And if I go on a consistent basis, which I try to, I notice a difference. I'm calmer, my spine is more upright and I feel taller. But what makes me feel even better—whenever I see Mr. Chow on that Citibank commercial with Ellen DeGeneres, his posture isn't that good.

12

CRANIALING

The 150 mg was starting to kick in and my head began to feel the way it did when I first got on 100 mg and 50 mg way back when. But physically, I wasn't so good. I was beginning to feel the side effects of the Zoloft, just as Dr. Tamm had initially warned me. The 50 mg and the 100 mg had both markedly decreased my sex drive, and the 150 mg all but killed it. The only saving grace was that Nancy was too busy brainstorming with Team Sitcom on the funniest possible quip for a surly neighbor to say right before a commercial break to notice.

Meanwhile, pain in my shoulders, upper back and neck was flaring up again. It didn't take much. Awkwardly holding a grocery bag, throwing a Frisbee, looking over my shoulder to merge. I'd been dealing with some degree of discomfort in those areas for decades, thanks to weight lifting and my street fight in that icy parking lot twenty-three years ago.

This time, I'd slept the wrong way on my neck and woke up in agony. I was barking at everybody: Nancy, my mechanic, the person who answers the phone at Supercuts. No wonder my mother is always so quick to snap; it's hard for the mind to relax when the body's always screaming at it. As the aches contract and close in, time is stretched so that a minute feels like ten and a half hour feels like a day. Impatience breeds. Even on 150 mg.

I needed relief and two or three ibuprofen did nothing. And since I didn't want to mess up my kidneys, as it says on the warning label, I didn't want to go up to four or five. So when I discovered Craniosacral therapy in a health journal at my dentist's office, I jumped at the chance to deplete my bank account even further. According to the magazine, it focused on "reducing tension and stress in the meningeal membrane and its fascial connections to enhance the functioning of the Craniosacral system, a fluid circulatory system that surrounds and protects the brain and spinal cord." Not going to win any Clio Awards, but worth a shot.

I made an appointment and was informed that the initial visit would run me $215. That seemed like a bargain to pay someone to "manipulate the bones of the head and spine and the membranes beneath the skull to allow free movement by the cerebrospinal fluid and balance energy fields."

As I walked into Craniosacral headquarters in downtown Los Angeles, an older, balding, ultra-stressed guy in a black T-shirt rudely bumped into me, with nary a glance or an "excuse me." Apparently he had the appointment ahead of me. He was one tense guy and looked as though he'd implode if he was kept in the waiting room a second past his scheduled time. I was hoping that wasn't going to be me in twenty-five years. I considered postponing my appointment and sneaking around in the parking lot so I could see what Oldie-But-Tensey looked like *after* his visit. If he was still a bundle of angst, then maybe this whole thing was a bad idea and I would just leave.

As I sat in the lobby, I noticed a collection of CDs for sale on the front counter. The cardboard display indicated that the soothing New Age music I was currently hearing was composed and produced by Dr. Whitehurst, the very doctor who would soon be treating me. The discs were $21.99 (plus tax), which seems like a lot of money to charge for a guy who already has a lucrative day job and drives a Lexus. For fucksakes, I could get the new Dylan album at Starbucks for half that. I wondered if, under any conditions, Blue Cross covered music.

As I listened to the instrumental mumbo jumbo ricocheting out of the cute little Bose speakers above my head, I hoped Whitehurst was a better doctor than musician. This stuff was unmelodic, monotonous drivel. The longer I waited, the more I wanted to buy up the entire display of CDs, including the one playing, and then go outside and run them all over with my Volvo.

Fifteen minutes later, Black-shirt guy emerged from the examination room. His harried walk had slowed to semi-harried and the scowl had been eased off his face. I would be staying. Although I really wished the receptionist took musical requests.

"Hi, I'm Dr. Whitehurst," said a slickly dressed fifty-year-old with jet-black hair. We shook hands and I followed him into a room that had a large maroon cushiony table with several smaller cushions protruding from the sides.

"So why are you here?"

I wanted to reply, "To hear some of the worst music on planet Earth." Instead I summed up my life.

"I'd like to relieve all the pain in my neck and upper back so I can be less tense and get off my medication before I hit 200 mg and I've tried everything. Zoloft, yoga, Kabbalah, anger management, sitting-still meditation, Tai Chi. I'm basically a tense guy on a deadline."

"Well, I think you'll be pleasantly surprised with this treatment." Then, in an instant, his smile turned into a scream. "Sheila!"

The receptionist who was minding the music warehouse up front entered carrying a pen and pad.

Whitehurst opened one of the cabinets and slid out a giant rectangular Lucite protractor.

"First we need to measure your neck's range of motion."

The giant protractor had a semicircle cut out from one of the sides where I could insert my head. I was instructed to bend my neck to the left, to the right, forward and back, then rotate it to the left and to the right. As I did, Whitehurst yelled out the corresponding numbers.

"Seventy degrees . . . sixty degrees . . . sixty-three . . . no, sixty-five degrees . . ." as Sheila eagerly recorded the data the way they do in a dentist's office to measure gum pockets.

"Are those good numbers?" I interrupted.

"No," Whitehurst shot back. "You were in a car accident, right?"

"No."

"Well, your neck should be able to turn ninety degrees in each direction. At least eighty-five."

Sheila looked sad as Whitehurst returned the giant protractor to its cabinet.

"Okay." Whitehurst motioned to me. "Why don't you lie down on this table, face up?" Seconds after I did so, another series of numbers was transferred from his mouth to Sheila's pad.

"Left ear an inch lower than the right . . . nose veers off to the right . . . left cheekbone a half inch too high . . ."

Thanks for the facial deformity update. Why not just come right out and call me ugly? Or maybe you can write a song about my uneven face for your next album. Oh, I forgot. None of your songs have lyrics. Or melodies for that matter.

"Do you grind your teeth?"

"I used to." In fact, when I first met Nancy that was one of our bonding moments. We both slept with mouth guards.

"Right part of jaw quarter of an inch lower than left."

Also, my right shoulder was much higher than my left, my hips were of varying heights, my left leg was shorter than my right, and my feet were flat. How had I ever managed to get laid?

Sheila packed up her pad and left the two of us alone as I sat up and contemplated diving out the window.

"We should talk about how many sessions you'll be coming in for," Whitehurst insisted. So far all you've done is mock and measure me. How about we complete the first visit and then discuss our future together?

"I'd prefer that—" But Whitehurst cut me off.

"I've been doing this type of work for sixteen years and I'd say there's a seventy-five percent chance of me helping you."

So only a twenty-five percent chance of me wasting my money.

"Listen, it all sounds good"—I tried to finish my thought—"I'd just like to—"

"I think we should start with two visits a week for six weeks and then take it from there."

"Look, I don't even know what you do."

"Of course. Well, after you see what I do, I think you'll be pleased."

I was starting to get agitated. This small talk was eating into my day and they only validated parking for an hour. After that it was $1.75 every fifteen minutes. I wasn't willing to pay another $7 an hour to listen to this desperate, insecure, greasy-haired Yanni wannabe.

"Great," I replied.

I noticed a framed Vector Point Cranial Therapy wall chart in back of him as he continued his sales pitch. The poster had a cartoonish profile of a skull covered in a series of dots. Each of the dots led directly to a specific organ: the colon, liver, pancreas, etc. In reality, we were all just fleshy puppets, controlled by a series of meridians that stretched from head to toe.

He had me lie down again on my back.

"Now, I want you to pull both of your feet back from the ankles while you inhale through your mouth and then exhale as you push them forward."

I began to deeply inhale and exhale while pumping my feet faster and faster and faster, as if I were hitting the gas and brakes of a car at the same time (which, incidentally, is dangerous) while Whitehurst pressed really hard on a series of spots on my head, spending no more than ten seconds in any one place—my cheekbones, behind my ears, under my jaw.

"What's the feet-pumping for?"

"It's called a Cranial-sacral pump. It's supposed to move your cerebrospinal fluids around."

"Supposed to?"

"Well, there's no proof that it does that, but that's what we think it does. We *wish* we had proof."

No wonder insurance didn't cover this.

"So exactly how is this supposed to help my neck and upper back?"

"I'm retraining the small muscles along the spine. By remote control!"

"You mean the pressure points on my skull?"

"Exactly!"

He then enthusiastically pushed both sides of my head together as if he were a human vise and my skull a two-by-four, which I'm pretty sure you should never do to a baby.

As he continued to press on areas of my face that had never been exposed to one-tenth the pressure he was applying, it felt weird, but it didn't hurt. He stopped pressing.

"Okay, now how do you feel?" he asked.

I sat up and I had markedly less pain in my neck and shoulders.

"Good."

He remeasured my ears. They had evened out. My cranium was cooperating.

"Your shoulders have evened out, too."

"Already?"

"Yes, but they'll probably snap back out of alignment without more visits. Ten more sessions and we'll get you as good as new."

"Ten?!" The parking alone would cost a fortune. "Let me think about it." Then after an awkward silence I added, "Are we done?"

"No. I need to strength-test your limbs."

As I remained on my back on the cushiony vinyl table I raised each of my limbs individually as Whitehurst pressed against them while I was told to resist his pressure.

"Your left leg is really weak. Let's see if we can fix that."

"Okay."

"First put both of your hands over your left eyebrow. I know it sounds odd but just do it."

I felt as if I were playing a game of face Twister.

He then pushed again on my left leg as I tried to resist his pressure. With my hands above my eyebrow, my leg was even weaker.

"Just as I thought," said Whitehurst, who then yanked a pair of rubber gloves out of his back pocket.

Okay . . . pumping my feet like a maniac and putting both hands over my left eyebrow were strange enough but when someone abruptly pulls out a couple of rubber gloves, that can't be a good thing.

I thought he was going to give me a prostate exam, of which I've had my fill. I don't know if there's anything more painful. To have some stranger with large hands ram a finger up your ass is bad enough when your prostate is healthy. To have some stranger with large hands ram a finger up your ass when your prostate is inflamed is intolerable. But Whitehurst didn't go anywhere near my ass.

"Open your mouth and relax your jaw, please."

He then shoved his gloved hand into various crevices inside my head, pressing on the inside of my facial bones, my hard palate and various other spots inside my mouth that only my tongue and some Turkish taffy had ever touched.

"Believe it or not, this'll strengthen that left leg of yours."

I couldn't answer. He had his hands in my mouth.

"Okay, let's test that leg again."

He removed his paws from the inside of my head and took off his gloves.

"Hands above the left eyebrow, please."

I again put both of my hands above my left eyebrow and raised my left leg as Whitehurst pushed down on it. It really was stronger! And I didn't think it was because he wasn't pushing on my leg as hard. This was indisputable.

"Pretty amazing, huh?" he bragged.

"Yes." I felt great. This was much better than a chiropractor.

"Okay, just one more thing. Open your mouth again."

Moments after I did, Whitehurst's magic gloves were back on and his fingers were pressing down on various parts of my interior skull. Then they started to drift near the back of my throat, flailing around like he was fishing for his car keys. And then . . . my head shot up like a catapult. I had thrown up all over him.

We looked at each other, equally disgusted. I was furious because he had hit my gag reflex, which I'm assuming wasn't supposed to happen. He was furious because I had ejected last night's chicken-pineapple curry onto his monogrammed dress shirt. I hadn't thrown up anything since I split a bottle of Smirnoff with Ronnie Lopez in eleventh grade. It didn't feel good.

"That wasn't supposed to happen, was it?" I queried.

"No, it wasn't."

"Well, your hand must've slipped."

"It didn't."

We each conveyed an unusual mixture of embarrassment and rage. It was bad enough throwing up in a parking lot in the middle of the night as a teenager in front of other throwing-up teenagers, but to propel my favorite Thai meal all over a guy I'd met less than an hour ago under 100-watt fluorescents was really uncomfortable and awkward. But I did the right thing. Had my head remained flat, I could have easily choked on my vomit.

Whitehurst trudged over to his desk and began blotting his shirt with tissues, fragments of which stuck to his clothes and made it look as if he had pineapple-y dandruff. He was extra miffed because it was only eleven-thirty and he probably didn't have another shirt to change into and would smell pungent for the remainder of his patients. I thought of offering him my sweatshirt, since I had a T-shirt underneath, but decided against it. Doctors and sweatshirts don't really belong together, unless they're out playing ball with their sons in a commercial.

The silence became painful. I didn't pay $215 for tension. My breath was hounding me and I had just run out of Listermint strips. You know your breath is really bad when your mouth is shut and you can still smell it. It's like after a workout when Nancy can smell my armpits through the tops of my shoulders.

Then, just as our emotions were about to boil over, Whitehurst and I acted as if nothing had happened—as if we both had just had really bad sex.

"So," he finally said, breaking the ice. "Let me give you your homework for next time."

"Let me guess: Don't eat dinner the night before?"

He fake-smiled, then showed me an isometric exercise where I'd press my left hand against the left side of my head while trying to bend my neck to the left. This would help to balance out my neck muscles so they wouldn't be fighting with each other. But that's the only exercise he dispensed. I'm sure he had others but was rationing them out to maximize my visits and his earning potential.

"And we should set something up for next week. I think I just had a cancellation Tuesday."

"Tuesday's great."

I followed him to the front desk and confirmed my new appointment with Sheila as Whitehurst stood behind me. Despite being closer to the exit, things felt even more awkward. I wish I could've just scampered out, but Sheila was in the process of running my credit card through the machine.

"Oh, Sheila," I bellowed. "Why don't you tack on a couple of Dr. Whitehurst's CDs." Then as I grabbed a pair of the discs from the display I turned to Whitehurst and added, "I really like your music." I don't know why I had to (a) bellow, (b) lie, or (c) buy more than one of his CDs, but I felt that two seemed more sincere and less patronizing, as if they were so entertaining that they'd make great gifts.

He seemed pleased.

I tossed the CDs into the trunk of my car and as soon as I got home I called Sheila and canceled my appointment. Then I brushed my teeth.

13

AYURVEDA-ING

"Ayurveda is not a licensed health care practice."

Those were the words at the top of the waiver form I was about to sign. I had driven several hours outside Los Angeles to get rid of some "ama." According to Ayurveda, which has been around for 5,000 years, disease is an imbalance in one's natural doshas caused by improper diet, poor digestion, negative emotions and stress, which subsequently leads to a buildup of toxins in the body called ama. I had reason to believe I had a lot of ama.

I sat in a wooden folding chair across from a light blue couch as Gregorian chants (which blew away Whitehurst's tunes) seeped out from one of the other rooms. The walls had but one lone tapestry—an elephant with a human body and lots of arms. If I angled my head properly, I could see a taco stand across the street from the nondescript office building I was in. Above my head was an assortment of diplomas from The American University of Complementary Medicine, Samra Oriental Medicine College, and The Acupuncture Committee. Individually, all three seemed rather pointless; collectively they seemed even more absurd.

Nearby there were also several stalks of bamboo in a vase, which pissed me off. Bamboo is supposed to be both lucky and tranquil but has quite the opposite effect on me. Besides not cleaning up after their dog, our next-door neighbors are abominably loud. So Nancy and I decided we needed to block out some of the sound from their yard with tall plants against our shared fence. We hired a landscaper through a friend of Nancy's, and the plant guy, Brad, suggested bamboo. The only hitch was that Brad, this little five-foot-one, ninety-five-pound man with the voice of a linebacker, didn't know what the fuck he was talking about. I shelled out over $1,300, and despite standing outside with a hose and hand-watering the stalks like a jackass for forty-five minutes every day as I was told, everything died within a month. Apparently it was the wrong kind of bamboo for our climate. We were bamboozled. That one's for Tai Chi Steve.

"Any treatments are not ment to replace prescribed medical treatments that the patient is undergoing."

"Ment"? Don't their computers have spell-check? Bad spelling has always irritated me but at least when using a Smith-Corona typewriter in the early '80s there was a shred of an excuse. There might not have been a dictionary nearby, or if there was, getting up to grab it was too much of a hassle. And that doesn't even address the laborious world of correction cartridges. But there's no longer a reason for bad spelling. Even the lamest computers in the world come with spell-check. In fact, when I spelled "spellcheck" without a hyphen, my computer magically added a red line under the word. What did these people think the red line under the word "ment" meant? That the word was resting on a tiny carpet? If they were this sloppy with their spelling, it didn't bode well for their being meticulous Ayurvedists.

"On a scale of 1–10, what is your energy today?"

It was probably a seven when I walked in but it had quickly escalated after being exposed to bamboo and the anti–spelling bee exhibit. I put 8.5 on the form.

"Clearly state three main health concerns."

I immediately wrote "Calm down" then stared into space, thinking of additional concerns. Although it seemed as if I had a lot of problems, I really only had one. After five minutes I couldn't think of anything else so I just wrote "Calm down" two more times.

"Is your elimination on the loose side or the hard side?"

Based on what? Compared with metamorphic rock it's kind

of loose but compared with the stuff inside a lava lamp—I'd be lying if I said it wasn't hard. I stopped overanalyzing and just put down "Normal." Which was more polite than "None of your business."

"Is your elimination feel complete?"

First of all, it's DOES! *Does* your elimination feel complete!!! Is your education feel complete? I felt like working out a deal with this place; I'd proof all of their literature and they'd Ayurveda me for free.

"Do you have any emotional, mental or psychological stress?"

Funny you should ask. And your collection of bad grammar and poor syntax has added to the pile.

After I'd answered another handful of questions, a bearded guy in his late thirties with wire-rimmed glasses introduced himself as Todd and told me to sit down next to him on the couch.

"We'll go over your questionnaire sheet later. First we're gonna take your pulse."

Todd propped my right arm up on a pillow and pressed his thumb down onto a vein on the inside of my right forearm, a few inches below my wrist. I'd had my pulse taken hundreds of times and was accustomed to this taking a minute, two minutes tops. Instead, we sat there in silence for much longer than that as he occasionally scribbled something on his clipboard with his free hand. He wasn't really writing anything, just scribbling. I glanced over at his clipboard and saw that there were three rows of nine figures of preprinted shapes that looked like orange wedges. I had no idea what the hell he was doing. He could have been bored and doodling for all I knew.

About ten minutes later, Todd still hadn't removed his thumb from my arm. I was getting antsy. I wondered if he had just spaced out and was thinking about the hole in his moccasins. Another few minutes passed. I couldn't wait until this was over. Then after six or seven more minutes, Todd released his hitchhiking finger and I thought it was.

"All right." He seemed even more exasperated and bored than me. "Let's get the other side now."

Todd and I switched places and he did the exact same thing on my left arm. This was tedious. I wanted a taco.

Another twenty minutes later, Todd's pad was completely covered in blue swirls and scrawls and his thumb was no longer glued to my body.

"All right." He seemed to have a favorite phrase for starting sentences. "Let's see what's going on inside of you." I thought he was going to look down my throat, in my ears or up my ass, but instead he just consulted his scribbles.

"All right, I bet that you never get headaches."

I didn't.

"I don't."

"And that you have a lot of neck and shoulder pain and quite a bit of joint pain."

That was dead-on! How the hell did he know that?

"Yeah!"

"And most of your stress is from the neck up."

"Absolutely! And you can tell all this stuff just from my pulse?"

"It's actually seven different pulses."

"I thought we only had one pulse."

"You do. I'm getting seven different readings by going to deeper and deeper levels."

"How do you go to different levels?"

"I press down a little harder each time."

This was magic. It was like holding down the "3" button in a department store elevator and knowing every item that would be at that floor. I still didn't understand, though. And he probably couldn't share his secret, unlike that table magic guy in Orlando telling me how he made the Queen of Hearts come out of Nancy's bra.

"All right." He went back to his notes. "You also have really dry skin."

That was true as well. In fact, when I was seventeen, my

hands became so dry from washing dishes at the Scupper that Dr. Torino told me I'd have to avoid using any water on my palms for a month. I wore rubber gloves at work and in the shower and used a waterless oatmeal paste to wash. This was starting to get weird.

"Each level is connected to different energy levels of the body. Some levels are connected to fat tissue, others to bone or nerves. We get all these readings and tabulate a Pitta-Vata reading."

"What's mine?"

"Your Pitta is three and your Vata is three."

"So that's pretty low."

"No, it's on a scale of one to three, not one to ten. Your Pitta-Vata is as high as it can go."

"Is that bad?"

"It's not good. All right, stick out your tongue."

As I did so, Todd leaned forward to get a closer look and I practically poked him in the eye with my giant mouth muscle. He then rapidly sketched something on another sheet on his clipboard, this one with a series of preprinted tongue shapes on it.

"All right, you have a series of red dots on the tip of your tongue . . ."

"Which I'm assuming isn't good. I mean, because of my bad Pitta-Vata scores."

"You're right. The red dots indicate fire and heat in your muscles. You don't need quite as much as you're carrying around."

"So now what?"

"We're gonna try to fix you."

"Good."

"A large portion of your stress is in your physiology, not just in your emotions. You're lucky. It's a self-feeding cycle, but we can deal with it."

"You mean that the stress in my brain is creating stress in my body, which then sends more stress up into my brain and then back down to my body again?"

"Something like that. Yeah."

I followed Todd down a long hallway into a kitchen with shelves filled with jars, spices and a bunch of yellow stuff. A white tapestry dangled from the ceiling. There were pots and pans scattered about and it looked as if a mad hippie scientist had been residing there.

Todd handed me a sheet of paper.

"All right, here's your new diet."

Diet? I hadn't come here to lose weight. And if this was so specialized, how did he spend forty minutes on my pulse and all of nine seconds putting together an indefinite meal plan?

"You can eat anything you want off this sheet whenever you want," he continued. "Stuff with an asterisk you can have once in a while, stuff with two asterisks you should only have in very small amounts."

"So anything without an asterisk I can eat a lot of?"

"Yep."

I looked at the list, which was broken up into fruits, vegetables, grains, meats, beans, nuts, seeds, sweeteners, spices, condiments, dairy, beverages and herb teas. After I read it for a second, Todd grabbed it back from me.

"All right, I want you to have half a glass a day of aloe vera juice, too," he said while circling that under the beverage category, then handing me back the sheet.

"And nothing cold. *Never* drink anything cold."

"Why not?"

"It's bad for your organs. Room-temperature or hot drinks only."

"What about wine?" I trembled.

"Only sulfite-free."

I looked under the beverage heading and began to get nauseated. Everything I liked to drink wasn't on the list. Everything I hated was. Apricot juice. Hated apricots. Cherry juice. Hated cherries. Grape juice. No thank you. Peach nectar. Pass. Orange juice and carrot juice, which I liked, each had two asterisks, which meant I could rarely have any. Cranberry juice, which I needed to drink for my prostate, wasn't even listed. The only thing I could even stomach was mango juice, and I doubt it would be as appealing un-cold. I had no idea what aloe vera juice tasted like but it couldn't be worse than prune juice (two asterisks, thankfully!).

I scanned the fruits and vegetables and was just as surprised. Lettuce had two asterisks, as did broccoli, carrots and kiwi. Any foods not listed—such as apples, pineapples and cucumbers—were forbidden. Even tomatoes weren't on the sheet, which meant I could never have them, even though, like cranberries, they were supposed to be essential for good prostate care. This diet was already turning into a *Sophie's Choice,* pitting one part of my body against another.

Todd grabbed the sheet back from me again.

"Let's work on your breakfast now. You like figs?" he asked.

"No. Hate 'em."

"Plums?"

"Nope."

"Prunes?"

"Won't touch 'em."

"Apricots?"

"No."

"Raisins? You must like raisins?"

"I'd rather die."

I started to get queasy. I was on the verge of another panic attack based solely on looking at a sheet of paper that contained words for things that I preferred not to eat. It was ironic that I had such an adverse reaction to so many of the foods on the list that were supposed to calm me down. In order to exorcise my demons I would be forced to eat stuff that frightened me.

"Okay, um . . ." Todd muttered as he developed a contingency plan on the fly. I'm sure he hadn't run into someone who hated so many foods. "You like berries?"

"Blue. No. Boysen. Uh-uh. Raspberries, yes. Blackberries, yes." I realized that none of these patterns even made sense, but whose food aversions do?

"Then I want you to mix a cup of blueberries . . ."

"I don't like blueberries."

"I meant blackberries."

"Okay."

". . . with some raspberries and a mango. That's your breakfast. But I don't want you to just cut everything up. I want you to mash it into a paste so it's like applesauce or baby food."

I didn't question the mashing command. I just assumed that since I wasn't big on chewing things, this was to aid my digestion. But he knew nothing of my chewing issues.

"What about bananas? Can I have bananas?"

"No bananas."

"Ever?"

"They're bad for people like you. So is anything spicy. Nothing spicy. Ever. If they have mild, you ask for 'mild, mild.'"

"What about sushi?"

"Once a week. At the most. And try to stick to the freshwater fish."

I liked spicy stuff and sushi and bananas. This Ayurveda guy was a culinary tyrant.

Then more problems flared up.

"Have you ever had ghee before?" (Note: the "h" is silent, the "g" is hard—like "Guy" if you're French.)

Before I could answer, he continued, "Ghee is a milk product."

He knew nothing of my milk issues, either.

"I get freaked out about milk. I haven't had any since I was six months old. I can't even put it in my cereal. I can't have milk." I began to sweat.

"It's not milk. It's more of a clarified butter."

That explanation didn't help any. I hated butter. I never put it on anything. And for taste reasons, not health reasons. Even as a child I ate my corn on the cob dry, my toast dry, my mashed potatoes dry. I was starting to turn as white as a glass of milk just thinking about this shit.

"All right," Todd continued. "I want you to take one tablespoon of ghee every morning on an empty stomach. Then wait a half hour before eating."

"You want me to eat clarified butter every morning?"

Now that I knew what it was, I couldn't even hear the word "ghee" without freaking out. I'd never be able to actually interact with it, especially on a daily basis. I was getting more and more nauseated. Despite 150 mg of Zoloft, I was helpless against milk product talk.

"It's good for you," he assured me. "A lot of the oils and bad stuff have already been removed."

I passed out.

When I awoke about ten minutes later, Todd was towering above me, relieved that he hadn't killed me with his talk of ghee.

"Are you all right?"

It was the first time he'd used those words at the end of a sentence.

"Not really."

It took me another fifteen minutes of heavy breathing and water drinking to get back to normal.

"All right, just stick a little in a shot glass in a microwave for twenty or thirty seconds and pretend it's medicine."

"Are you talking about the ghee again?"

"Yes."

"Please don't. I'll need to make a decision about the ghee on my own. I'll keep you posted about the ghee."

My Pitta-Vata was probably both fives now.

Soon after, Todd began mixing a bunch of herbs into a large jar, which he then handed to me.

"Put a teaspoon of this into hot water and drink two cups a day."

"Is there any ghee in that?"

"No."

I took the jar, which looked as if it were filled with dirt.

"Drink one cup after breakfast and one after lunch."

Todd then took my credit card and added everything up: $235 for the pulse reading and the dietary guide, $53 for the herbs.

"Fifty-three dollars?" I asked.

"It would cost you over a hundred twenty in a store."

Then charge even more, idiot.

"Can I ask you a question . . ."

"Sure."

"Where would I get some ghee . . . y'know . . . if I *were* interested?"

"We sell it here. In fact the raw organic stuff is hard to find in stores and it tastes way better than the nonorganic."

I sighed overdramatically and agreed to some ghee. If I was going to try this Ayurveda, I didn't want to skip a key ingredient.

The ghee came in a clear Mason jar, had a rich yellow custardy color and was $25. However, on the way home it would not be riding up front with me.

"All right, you'll come back next month and we'll see how you're doing."

"All right."

The first thing I noticed as I walked down the aisles of the health food store with my empty cart was that blackberries and raspberries are really expensive. And I don't even mean the organic kind. I'm talking about the cheap stuff filled with pesticides and chemicals and perhaps a stubborn bug or two. The blackberries were $4.99 and the raspberries $5.99—and for tiny baskets. And mangos weren't cheap either: $2.49 each. The aloe vera juice was almost $10 for a small bottle that would probably last a week if I was lucky. But according to the label it would "support my immune and gastrointestinal systems, aid digestion, give muscle and joint support, and help maintain healthy gums." Okay, maybe the aloe vera juice was a bargain—but it still wouldn't offset the mango/berry expenditure. Even the almond oil was $12.99 for a toothpaste-sized container. Oh, I didn't even mention the almond oil. I was supposed to have Nancy massage some into my scalp for fifteen to twenty minutes every morning as soon as I woke up. This apparently would serve the dual role of helping me to relax and making Nancy resent me. Asking someone to take up twenty valuable minutes of her morning time before work (not to mention another five minutes to wash all the oil off her hands) seemed insane. But once I passed the almond oil aisle, I couldn't resist. I would strive for completeness, even if it meant doing my own massaging.

I'm not really big on putting things in my hair, either. My brother started losing his when he was nineteen. I'm forty-two and I still have it all, which I attribute to three things. (a) I never blow-dry my hair. I did it on the very first day of eighth grade and not only did it make my hair look really poofy—even by late-'70s standards—but it felt like I was napalming every strand. Blasts of heat an inch away from your follicles can't possibly be good for your hair. (b) No caffeine. Since I'm a bundle of nerves, my body doesn't need it anyway, and as a teenager I remember reading a study that linked caffeine to hair loss. I'm not sure if it's true, but I'm not taking any chances. (c) Sweat. Every time I miss a week or two of exercising, I notice that my hair doesn't grow as fast, if at all. On the other hand, when I work out every day, it sprouts out of my skull like a fern. This theory I'm adamant about. Exercise + sweating = good head circulation and more nutrients to your hair. (And yes, my mother's father died with a full head of hair; however, how would that explain my brother's deficiency?) Also, I never wear hats. They restrict circulation. The point is, the almond oil purchase showed just how much I meant business.

The next morning, I began my new way of life.

I stood over the kitchen counter, slowly unscrewed the Mason jar and stared at the ghee for about a minute. Then I frantically screwed the top of the jar back on and took a break. The ghee had a popcorn-buttery smell and the consistency of a lemon

Italian ice. I went upstairs, popped a Zoloft (which I usually take at lunchtime but I needed a little immediate help) and went back downstairs to give it another try.

I recalled seeing the title "Ghee Artisan" among Todd's many Ayurvedian accomplishments on his business card and it suddenly struck me how odd that was. I didn't think getting ghee into a Mason jar was exactly worthy of the moniker "Artisan." I think an ice sculptor is worthy of being called a "Water Artisan," but I'm not sure every digestible item warrants such hyperbole.

I lined up several glasses of water, held my breath as if trying to cure hiccups and reopened the ghee jar. I scooped out a tablespoonful, stuffed it into my mouth and drank my designated water. I considered following that with a few shots of scotch but I didn't want to get in the habit of drinking hard liquor at seven-thirty in the morning. Instead, I spit into my sink about fifteen times. No wonder ghee isn't more popular—it tastes horrible. Although I didn't eat red meat, I vowed that if I were to go to a wedding and the dinner options were baby antelope or the ghee platter, I'd opt for the former.

Since I had twenty-eight more minutes to kill before I was permitted to eat my breakfast, I decided to start preparing it. I was not a kitchen person. We order takeout pretty much every day and the only thing Nancy can cook is brisket, which, Ayurveda or no Ayurveda, I can't eat. The only time I'm ever in the kitchen is to get a real fork if a prong on the plastic one cracks or to cork up red wine.

I immediately had a cantankerous relationship with the mango. This was turning out to be a pain in the ass. No wonder people go out for breakfast. There's no easy way to separate the mango-y edible part from the unruly pit and the series of random abrupt curves lead to a lot of jarring knife maneuvers. Damn, was this messy! And dangerous.

Then the blackberries and raspberries had to be washed and thrown together with the mango and smushed into a paste, as per Todd. I would not be smushing my food into a paste. Let my stomach do that; that's its job. I poured myself a glass of aloe vera juice, which looked like tinted water, and stared at it as I continued fasting until my half hour was up.

Breakfast was delicious. But time-consuming. And money-consuming. About $9.50 a day, way more expensive than my customary banana and muffin. And that didn't even include the prorated price of the herbs for my post-meal tea. Or the ghee. I was getting stressed just figuring out how I could afford to eat this way. I would have to suck it up for a month and see how I felt.

The next morning I woke up and the changes were unbelievable: I was calm, composed and a host of other words I could thesaurus but was way too relaxed to bother with. The transformation was instant, profound and startling. I assumed it was just my body getting used to something new, like when I hadn't worked out in a month because of walking pneumonia but then did a set of bench presses and my chest was sore for the next eleven days.

But it wasn't. I remained relaxed, levelheaded, balanced. It was a miracle. What was responsible for these resounding results? Was it the ghee? The herbs in the tea? The pricey new foods that were better suited to my body? The old foods I had eliminated from my diet that weren't good for my body? Sure, a banana, carrot juice and broiled salmon were healthy on paper, but apparently had adverse effects on my body-type/personality-type/energy-type. And, because I was a creature of habit, I'd been ingesting the same group of foods day after day, year after year, so the mistakes I had been making were like compounding interest, growing exponentially and building up in my body.

I remembered reading a study several years ago that found a correlation between a higher intake of omega-3 fatty acids and lower murder rates. Not that my violent tendencies approach the killing level, but I bet very few murderers are mellow while on the clock. The infamous "Twinkie Defense" was starting to make sense. Maybe my diet was ultimately responsible for my erratic behavior. After all, the flood of fast food I consumed growing up was the healthy part of my eating regimen compared with my daily candy intake—Pixy Sticks, SweeTarts, Chuckles, Razzles, Jaw Breakers, Atomic Fireballs, Sugar Daddies and those candy buttons that you yank off wax paper. Because of my mother's illness and a lack of eating supervision, I had lived my teenage years as if every day were Halloween. True, I hadn't had candy in my twenties and thirties, but that adolescent decade of sugar gorging definitely could've impeded my path to calm.

Regardless, I was ecstatic. This Ayurveda stuff could put the Zoloft people out of business. Okay, probably not, because frankly, most Westerners are cynical and skeptical of any treatment by anyone not dressed in white with a stethoscope around his neck. Besides, just swallowing a pill is much easier than going shopping—which, whenever I was in a supermarket chain, consisted of me walking up and down the aisles like a zombie in search of something that wouldn't mess up my Pitta-Vata. . . . Can't eat that . . . can't eat that . . . not on list . . . damn it! . . . I'm starving . . . mango-pineapple juice . . . *must be only mango* . . . must purchase pineapple filter or invent one if it doesn't exist . . . help!!! The only other downside was that the herbs in the tea stained my teeth. But I rationalized that this would only make Orange Juice Carton Face more intimidating—if I ever even used it again.

Anyway, the results for me were indisputable.

Nancy noticed a huge transformation, too. And I in her. The mellower I became, the more stressed she got as her work hours started including weekends. She wanted to go to Ayurveda, too, but didn't have the time to drive two hours each way. I did some research and found an Indian guy who sporadically visits the Valley for consultations.

At her Ayurvedic session Nancy was told she had kidney stress, bladder trouble, potential colon ills, sensitive mucous membranes and the number of days until her next period. "The guy was amazing!" Nancy said in astonishment. "I mean, I didn't even tell him a thing about myself or fill out one sheet of paper. And he knew I peed a lot!"

But since Nancy went to a different place and her body type was different (Vata, with a little Pitta, whatever that means), her solutions were different. She told me the following as I was kneeling in our driveway, smashing my prescribed weekly coconut with a hammer.

"I'm supposed to drink a half gallon of water with grated ginger in it every day and eat barley with cinnamon for breakfast."

"I'm supposed to not do that."

"And he told me to make a paste out of turmeric and honey for my mucous problem and lick it off a spoon before I go to bed."

I was jealous because that sounded good and ghee sucked.

"I'm also supposed to buy special supplements online."

"Did he give you a list of things you could and couldn't eat?"

"Yes. Let's make a copy before I lose it."

"Can you have sushi?"

"No," she answered glumly. "But I'm allowed to eat spicy foods!"

"I can't eat anything spicy," I said sadly. "But you can still have avocado, right?" Nancy makes killer guacamole.

She scanned her dietary sheet for the answer.

"No. Not on here. Can you have brown rice? I'm supposed to eat a lot of brown rice."

"Two asterisks, so very little. Mangos?"

"No sweet fruits."

"Almond oil on scalp?"

"Sesame oil on shoulders."

"Will we ever share a meal again?"

"Probably not."

Although, through the grace of God, we both had asparagus on our sheets.

After thirty days I felt better than I ever had in my life and went back for my scheduled Pitta-Vata reanalysis.

o o o

Todd greeted me right in front of the bamboo—which miraculously no longer stirred up hostile memories.

"All right." He had on a green Izod shirt and had trimmed his beard. "How'd it go?"

"I feel amazing. I'm calm, relaxed, my colon doesn't palpitate like a second heartbeat. Even my joints don't crack as loudly as they used to."

"You take the ghee?"

"Yeah. I got used to it."

"Did you heat it up?"

"Nah. Just ate it right off the spoon."

"It tastes better if you heat it up."

"It's easier to just eat out of the jar. I wanted to spend as little time with it as possible. Can we please stop talking about ghee?"

"All right! I forgot. C'mon, let's check out your Pitta-Vata again."

We went back to the couch area and he proceeded to take lengthy readings on both wrists. My Pitta had dropped from a high three to a high two, and my Vata had gone down to one. And my surface Vata wasn't even noticeable anymore. Don't worry if you're confused; I still am. But I felt fantastic.

"All right! These results are great!" It was the most excited I had ever seen Todd.

"I still don't really get this whole Pitta-Vata thing."

"All right, the Pitta is more reactiveness and aggression. The Vata is more about sensitivity and anxiety."

"So the road rage is Pitta and the panic attacks—like the one I had here last month—is Vata?"

"Sure."

"So what's in the herb jar that I make the tea with?"

"You've probably never heard of any of it."

"I probably have," I said, all braggy and balanced.

He proceeded to jot down what he had included in my custom-made brew.

Gokshura
Manjistha
Amalaki
Bhumyamalaki
Chairata
Gugulu
Varisa Rochana
Jatamansi
Tagara

He was right. I had never heard of any of these things. But frankly, I didn't care if there was rabbit shit in my tea as long as I felt this good.

Since my Ayurvedic experience had been far better than expected, I signed up for the deluxe package for another $400. I didn't know the specifics of what it entailed. I was about to find out.

Todd told me to take off my clothes so I could get a special massage to open my pores and have the exact same nutrients that I had in my tea thrust into every crevice of my body. Now, unless I'm home alone, I'm not wild about being naked. (Yes, in my twenties I had no problem standing in front of strangers while wearing a Speedo and flexing, but the Speedo makes a big difference.) Actually, I wasn't completely naked. I was given a small white hand towel and told to place it vertically between my legs, which made me feel like a miniature sumo wrestler.

I wasn't used to a masseur. In fact, I'd rather have a really lame massage by a female than an awesome one by a male. I don't like the rough hands. Frankly, I could do without having a man touch me for the rest of my life. I think my dad and I have hugged once and I hated all six seconds of it. I'm not even comfortable shaking hands. So right off the bat, there was this odd dichotomy of having things done to my body designed to help me relax that just made me more tense.

After twenty non-blissful minutes of Todd rubbing the mudlike paste onto my back and legs, he told me to flip over and I did, clutching the mini-towel in hopes that it would cling to my groin. I was uptight enough while I was facedown staring at the ground, but now I'd be making occasional eye contact with the guy I'd just paid to put his hands all over me. I vowed to pretend I was asleep and keep my eyes shut until this madness was over. The good news was, at least he wasn't chatty. Todd put some dark paste on my face and moved down to my pectorals, where it seemed he was spending just a *little* too long rubbing my nipple area.

I opened my eyes about a millimeter and peeked over at Todd and then I noticed it. Todd had a hard-on. The only other possible explanation was that it was flaccid but gigantic. Either way, it was creepy. I had gone from uncomfortable to terrified. My body was tensing up so much that I wouldn't have been surprised if he thought rigor mortis was setting in.

I had to get the hell out of here! I wished there was some kind of nurse's button they have in hospitals that I could push that said "Okay, put your dick back between your legs, I've had enough male nipple rubbing!" But there wasn't. Had I not been naked and covered in mud, I might have just sprinted off. Instead, I cleared my throat to not so subtly notify Todd that he was going over the line, but he either didn't hear me or thought I was clearing my throat for medicinal purposes. The only saving grace at the moment was that I didn't remember seeing "cock" on my list of foods I could eat.

Maybe I'm a homophobe. My introduction to the gay community was rather jarring. I'd never even met a gay person until my first night of freshman year in college. My roommate, Ross, was overtly out of the closet and I was oblivious. I just thought people from western Massachusetts acted a little differently from Long Islanders. Ross was funny, polite and as good a roommate as I've ever had in or out of college; nonetheless, I was still nervous that he would spoon me in the middle of the night. I assumed this because all of his friends used to blatantly hit on me, but, in hindsight, only because they delighted in how uncomfortable it made me.

Then the unthinkable happened. Todd leaned over to massage the far side of my body and his—well, I'd like to think it was a pen in his pocket, but it wasn't—poked me in the cheek. It was like when a busty hairstylist leans over and her breasts rub against you. But that's fun. This wasn't.

"What the fuck!" I finally said. This was now officially the antithesis of relaxing.

"Oh, sorry."

Then he backed up a quarter of an inch. Now it was like that game you played with your siblings where they said "Stop touching me!" and you'd wave your hands millimeters away from their faces while announcing "I'm not touching you!" because *technically* you weren't. But it's actually even more annoying than being touched.

I was going to shoot him an Orange Juice Carton Face but feared that under my mud mask it would be unrecognizable or look like I was happy. So I merely changed the subject, hoping that the sound of my voice and a barrage of questions would turn him off.

"So . . . what's next . . . after this?"

"The hot box."

At least it wasn't called the rape box. I wished I'd just come back for a simple pulse reevaluation. Why did I have to take it this far? I wasn't even a spa fan when they were reasonably priced and I didn't have a strange man's dick trying to puncture my cheek.

I gingerly stepped off the massage table and followed Todd down a hallway to another small room that housed the hot box. I was uncomfortable and tense horizontally, but far worse when vertical and 97 percent naked following somebody down a hallway. Why couldn't he have just told me where to go and I'd meet him there? The place wasn't all that big and I'm really good at following directions. Give me a little space, ghee pusher!

Meanwhile, Todd acted as if the "trying to play groin-pool with my skull" was a normal part of his day. I was still mortified. Although my body was completely coated with the mud-like substance, I pushed the towel into my groin area with maximum force to retain a smattering of dignity. I would not let another man see my penis. For crying out loud, *I* didn't even want to see my penis. I've even considered keeping a piece of electrician's tape over it like when they blacked out the guys' privates in old porn magazines.

I followed Todd inside another room, where he propped open the lid of a small wooden crate and told me to sit inside it. Todd politely looked away, but that did nothing to quell my discomfort. Since my rear was completely bare, I backed into it as if I were a woman with a large sweater tied around her waist who didn't want anyone noticing her enormous ass.

I sat down, still naked and covered in mud, still clutching my small white towel to my groin, on a slab of wood covered with a beach towel. It was instantly sweltering. Then Todd closed the lid as I maneuvered my head through the hole in the top. For the next hour, I had no access to my face. I didn't like that. That's just one of many reasons I was never able to play guitar live. Too many twitches and itches. I'd have to stop and scratch my chin or nose every three chords. I can't even have a five o'clock shadow, let alone a beard. If I'm not clean-shaven, I touch my face incessantly. If I were an actor and really needed facial hair for a role, I'd have to wear a giant cone around my neck like a dog to prevent me from stroking my stubble. Maybe having my face estranged from the rest of my body would be a good thing. Maybe this would teach them both a lesson. It made me think of *Boxing Helena* starring Lara Flynn Boyle or that other girl from *Twin Peaks*. Whoever it was, I felt like her.

Every ten minutes or so, Todd would stop by and hold a small cup of water with a straw near my mouth. I was half-expecting him to tease me with the straw and make me bob and work for it, as if I were giving a blow job. I'm glad he didn't. While sweating, I made an agreement with myself to only look at him from the chest up. As far as I was concerned, he no longer had a lower body and was just the top part of a genie, floating in space.

After an hour of sweating toxins out of my system, I was instructed to get up and commute yet again—with my tiny towel, which had apparently gotten tinier from shrinking inside the hot box. Part of me was thinking of lying and telling him I was a doctor and that one of my patients had just paged me and there was a medical emergency and I had to go and thank you very much for everything. But (a) I wasn't a doctor and (b) naked people don't carry pagers.

I went into another room and was told to lie on another table, this one much lower to the ground. And the tenser I got, the more relaxed Todd became, probably because he enjoyed seeing me squirm.

"Okay," said Todd matter-of-factly. "Now I'm going to drip some hot oil on your forehead."

I thought this was to punish me, but apparently it was just another relaxation technique. So for the next thirty minutes hot oil dripped onto my forehead from a brass urn. Oil hot enough to cook an otter with. At first it felt like being tortured but I soon fell into a deep sleep, and I was later told that my legs and arms were twitching violently.

"All right! That's good. It means the stress is leaving your body."

When I woke up, it was the first time I felt relaxed since being poked. I was finally in a state of bliss. As I ran my fingers across my face, my hands didn't even recognize the skin. My entire body felt cleansed and energized. The herbs had produced the identical result that ingesting them accomplished. This was good. I couldn't wait to tell Nancy.

"Now, just sit here and relax. I'll be back in ten minutes."

When Todd returned, he was holding up a clear plastic bag

filled with dark green oily fluids, as if he had just caught a large trout.

"All right, I have an enema for you now."

Uh-oh.

"An enema?"

"Yes. Have you ever had one before?"

"It's been a while."

"Well, it's really good for your colon. Now, just roll over on your side, straighten the bottom leg and bend the top one and let me just slip it in there for you."

No fucking way this guy was gonna put something up my ass. I rolled back over onto my spine. I was in charge of my own ass.

"I . . . I'll do it," I stammered.

I then pretended that I was four years old and taking my temperature with a rectal thermometer and I stuck the plastic tube in as Todd jiggered with the bag so there'd be a constant stream of liquids flowing. There was a parade of silence while all of the green mineral-y stuff moved from the plastic, down the tube and into my colon. When the bag was empty, Todd spoke.

"All right, now lie flat on your back and see if you can hold all the fluids inside you for fifteen or twenty minutes. You think you can do that?"

I had no idea. It's not like I'd been training for the big enema competition.

"Sure."

"All right! Then you can shower off and get dressed." Todd was all business now. "All right. You did great!"

It seemed that this ordeal was wrapping up.

"We advise everyone to affix a panty shield to their underwear. You're gonna drip out of there for at least the next couple hours."

"Panty shields?"

"We have some in the bathroom. Just peel back the wings and stick it to the inside of your boxers . . . or briefs . . . or whatever."

Then Todd and I shook hands and he left me alone.

After showering and dressing, I took a deep breath, walked out of the building with a winged panty shield stuck to my boxers and had green mineral-y stuff dripping out of my ass for the next five hours, three of which were during rush hour. Other than that, I felt pretty damn good.

14

KNITTING

"That mud bath I had yesterday was unbelievable!" I said, eating a piece of asparagus with some mung beans.

"Good for you!" Nancy snapped resentfully. As a magazine writer I should have been jealous of her network sitcom job; instead she was jealous of my quest for calm.

I barely saw Nancy anymore thanks to her demanding work schedule. And between my taking 75 percent of the maximum recommended dose of Zoloft and her never being home, sex was starting to feel nostalgic. Even masturbation for healthy prostate care wasn't happening.

"How come we're not having sex anymore?" she queried.

"Because on the rare occasion I'm horny, you're either at work, home doing work for work, or asleep having nightmares about work."

"But you still find me attractive?"

"Of course! I just find 150 mg of Zoloft more attractive. But the Ayurveda is really working, so I'll drop back down to 100 mg and we can start having sex again."

"Good! Did you make an appointment with Dr. Tamm?"

"No, but I know what I'm doing. And if my hands start to itch again he'll be the first guy I call," I defiantly replied, as I accidentally ate some of Nancy's barley, which I promptly spit out into a napkin since it was forbidden under my Ayurvedic manifesto.

"But don't you need a new prescription?"

"Nah. I've got all kinds of samples I've been storing up. All it takes is some simple math and my pill cutter."

Then our smoke detector went off and Nancy jumped to attention, realizing she'd forgotten about her mana bread.

"Dammit! Our toaster sucks!"

"Then we'll get a new one. It's not worth getting upset over."

"Yes, it is! What's going on? You're the calm one now!"

"Well," I said, noticing that the microwave clock read 5:53. "I should get going or I'm gonna be late." Plus, in two minutes I'd be forced to stare at the clock for another minute.

When Nancy's friend Paula heard about my commitment to calming down, she suggested I try knitting. It had helped her deal with a new baby, a divorce and an ill sister. She took her knitting needles on airplanes, to restaurants, meetings, waiting rooms, everywhere. I was torn. "A guy doesn't knit!" I yelled internally at myself. "But I've never seen a tense knitter," another part of me yelled back so only I could hear it. I rationalized that if this didn't help me calm down, I'd at least have some leg warmers or a pot holder to show for my trouble.

When I was in high school and had to choose electives, all the other kids were taking metal shop and auto repair, but my mother suggested I take home economics so I could learn important day-to-day things, like sewing. That Nancy's really a lucky duck. Whenever one of her shirts needs a button, I sew the shit out of it. By hand, mind you. Over the course of our marriage, I've probably saved us nearly twenty dollars in sewing costs. Sewing and knitting seemed like close cousins.

Paula told me about a local beginners' class and I eagerly signed up. I assumed knitting would de-stress me in much the same way as Tai Chi, in that the monotonous repetitiveness would take my concentration away from the remainder of life. For $49, I'd be entitled to a pair of two-hour sessions, yarn, knitting needles, plus drinks and snacks. I had just missed the Mittens Class held on the nineteenth and twentieth. Which kind of bummed me out, but I rationalized that I shouldn't box myself in and be known for only one type of garment, so the standard beginners' group I signed up for would be for the best. Unless you're under ten or in an ice cream eating contest, you've got no business wearing mittens anyway.

As my Volvo and I repeatedly circled the block, I searched for a Learning Annex–type place but all I saw was a row of stores. After eight laps around, it dawned on me that the class would be held inside one of them. Probably the place that had lots of yarn and woolly things in the window.

I walked in ten minutes late and stressed because of it. I think the last time I was ten minutes late for anything was when I was trying to be a half hour late for a friend who was always an hour late. The store was filled with bright fluorescent lights to illuminate the high-end products such as yak wool area rugs, llama wool halter tops and dehaired goat wool socks. The Filipino cashier looked completely shocked to see a man in the store. It was as if I'd just walked into her bathroom stall.

I approached the cash register.

"Hi, I spoke with Cyndi on the phone."

"About?"

"The knitting class."

"Oh. The knitting class. Yes, I'm sorry. It's straight back, to the left."

I nodded and walked off.

There were six women gathered around a glass coffee table, no one older than forty. Knitting. Some had large things that may very well have grown up to be blankets; some had what looked like the arm of a sweater; others had barely enough yarn to make a bracelet. As I got within earshot of the group, the first words I heard were:

"A scarf can *never* be too wide."

I wanted to yell out, "Amen, sisters!"

I said hello to my fellow knitters and received a few hi's back, although no one bothered to look up from her needles. There was an assortment of decent-looking food: crackers, fancy cheeses, raspberries and several bottles of wine. Upon making eye contact with the plate, I promptly stuffed three raspberries in my mouth. I was psyched that I wouldn't have to stray from my Ayurvedic diet. I was allowed to eat all the raspberries I wanted.

Then Cyndi magically appeared from a back room. She had straight bleached-blond hair, was in her late forties and not wearing anything made of wool.

"Hi, I'm Cyndi. You must be the gentleman I spoke with on the phone."

I nodded. My mouth was filled with raspberries.

This was strange. The class was actually in plain view of all the customers. People could hypothetically walk in off the street and heckle my knitting. I was self-conscious enough as it was. I didn't like being out in the open like this. Plus, everyone was working so assiduously that I felt as if I were part of the world's most overt sweatshop.

"Well, why don't you have a seat and I'll help you get started."

I sat between a heavyset woman who was about halfway done with a cardigan and a sad-looking twenty-four-year-old who looked as if she had just gotten her hair cut really really short that morning but didn't mean for it to be quite that short.

"I've never knitted before."

"Oh, it's easy," said Cardigan gal.

"Okay, let's pick out a color or two," said Cyndi as she held several balls of yarn in front of me. I selected the dark blue.

"We don't often have men in here," she added.

"Oh, really," I said with mock surprise.

"Now, what we're going to do first is create a tail, which should be one and a half times the length of your arm."

"Sounds good."

"Now let's make a slipknot toward the top of the tail. Like this!" She demonstrated and then quickly undid her work so I'd be starting from scratch.

I kept tying regular knots instead. I was already in over my head.

"Didn't you ever make a slipknot in the Cub Scouts or something?"

"My brother did, but it probably wasn't under this much pressure."

"Would you like a glass of wine?"

I was sure that every bottle on the table had sulfites—forbidden by my Ayurvedic diet—but I needed to relax. Nancy would have also been torn here; she was allowed sulfites[7] but couldn't have raspberries. "Sure."

"Red or white?"

"Surprise me."

Cyndi poured me a hearty glass of merlot, tied a slipknot for me and resumed her lesson.

"Now we're going to learn how to cast on."

"Excellent," I said as I took a mountainous slurp from my giant glass. Damn. This stuff was incredible. Sulfites are delicious. And ghee sucks. I had it all backward.

"You can put down the other needle. We'll only be using one for now."

I sneaked in another sip as I stuck the second needle back in the small paper bag I'd been given.

Cyndi demonstrated as she spoke. "What you want to do is take the tail end and wind it around your left thumb, then wrap the yarn over your left index finger so your hand is in a gun shape."

I grabbed another raspberry and nodded.

"Then insert the needle—which is in your right hand—upward into the loop and your thumb and then bring it back from the index finger side and then pull your thumb back to tighten the loop on the needle. Here. Now you try."

I attempted, but it was as awkward as my trying to hold a fork as a teenager. I kept screwing up and Cyndi kept on undoing all of my work and restarting the process herself.

---

7. I was soon to learn at my local liquor store that ALL WINE contains sulfites. Mr. Cock-in-the-Cheek ment to only drink wine with NO ADDED SULFITES, aka organic wine.

"I'm going to leave you alone for a bit and work with these other students, but I think you're getting it."

I think you're lying.

"Okay."

I took another gulp of wine for inspiration. Then I stared intently at my needle and yarn and continued my cast-ons while I listened to some of the other knitters' conversations.

"Courtney, why are you all dressed up tonight?"

"I'm going to see Counting Crows."

"They were just on Leno."

"I can't stay up that late."

"You could tape it."

"I'd never catch up on everything."

"I can't believe Leno's quitting."

"Shut up!"

"You didn't know? Conan O'Brien is replacing him in 2013 or something."

"Conan is so tall."

"Yeah. He is."

"And Jay has that chin."

"Yeah. He does."

A new knitter straggled in with a baby.

"Sooo adorable."

"I know! Isn't she!"

"She really is," I piped in without looking up to see if she was.

"Y'know *Emily* is pregnant!"

"You are?"

"I am!"

"How far along?"

"Just ten weeks."

"You're in for the ride of your life!"

Did groups of guys talking seem this boring to women? I felt as if I were listening to 3-D versions of every meaningless cell phone call I've ever heard, only this time I had to hear both ends of the conversation.

I did about forty or fifty cast-ons before Cyndi returned.

"Oooh . . . okay. These are not *exactly* what we wanted. You're splitting the yarn on some of these and the others are just . . . um . . . wrong."

She again yanked apart all my work and started fresh for me. Meanwhile, I grabbed another fistful of raspberries and quaffed down some more merlot. I was starting to get buzzed.

I didn't understand how this was relaxing. Maybe compared to dealing with crying babies and racing toward menopause it was. Maybe compared to going through a divorce it was. Maybe compared to having a shiv stuck into your lungs it was. Perhaps I simply needed to amp up the stresses in my life and then I'd appreciate the true grandeur of yarn manipulation.

Once Cyndi did twenty cast-ons for me—in about eighteen seconds—it was time to remove the second needle from my little brown bag. I don't know what made her think I was ready to double the number of needles. I sucked with one. This couldn't possibly be easier than casting on. And I was right. I watched Cyndi demonstrate as the yarn magically wrapped around her fingers, through other fingers, and back out again like a Rube Goldberg drawing. It was actually pretty cool watching her do it. I felt like a cat being teased with a piece of string. *This* was relaxing.

"Ah, you finished your wine. Would you like another glass?"

"Sure!" If this whole knitting thing wasn't going to pan out, I was at least planning on drinking $49 worth of 2003 Kendall-Jackson.

"Now *you* try," she said while mercifully filling my glass to the top.

I picked up both needles and felt completely helpless. I tried to follow the instructions I had just received, but my hands seemed to have their own agenda. It was as if I were attempting to eat a single grain of rice with a set of chopsticks. Had Cyndi stabbed me with my knitting needles I wouldn't have pressed charges. She would have done us both a favor.

I repeated about ten or twelve knit stitches and thought I

was at least in the ballpark. Then I discovered otherwise, as Cyndi yanked all of my equipment out of my hands.

"You've just repeated the wrong stitch a dozen times."

"Oh," I apologized.

"And even if they were correct, you're pulling them way too tight, anyway."

"Whoops."

"Now WATCH ME *very carefully* this time."

I did, but once again the string of wool was zipping around everywhere and even my eyes couldn't keep up, let alone my brain and hands. If there were a knitting final I would definitely need to cheat off someone.

"Got it?"

"I think so."

"Okay, I'll be back in a few minutes to check up on you again."

Then Cyndi was off to help the gifted knitters.

I noticed that Van Morrison music had begun emerging from the speakers. It wasn't "Moondance" or that other famous song . . . which made me realize that he's lucky to have two famous songs. "I fucking hate that drunk!" I said to myself as I gulped some more wine. Then one of the other knitters reached for the last raspberry, but my fingers got there first. The hell with knitting. Scrapping for food was a far more valuable skill.

I continued my little project and hoped that when Cyndi returned she would be pleased and I wouldn't get yelled at. I didn't even actually know what I was trying to make. And she hadn't even asked. I began to think of odd things to knit: a football helmet, a saddle for an alpaca, a tent to cover a house when it's being de-termited. Perhaps a giant quilt that said "Thank God for Merlot and Sulfites!"

I took my mind off my knitting and listened to what the ladies had to say.

"I just got back from Toronto."

"How was it?"

"Too cold."

Then don't go. It's Toronto, you idiot!

"I mean, if it's gonna be *that* cold, I at least want some snow."

"I totally agree! Canada should always have snow. Otherwise, why bother to go there?"

"I like the snow."

"Snow is really fun."

"I like to ski."

"Oh, skiing is *really* fun!"

I'd changed my mind. Now I would knit myself a pair of earplugs.

Cyndi returned, reexamined the birth of my potential catheter warmer and yanked it apart like a man tearing a phone book in half.

"Okay! I want you to read the handouts this week and practice, practice, practice."

Hey, you know what rhymes with "knit"? Quit.

"Sure. I'll practice a lot."

"And we'll see you next Wednesday."

"Yep."

"It really is easy once you get the hang of it," said Cardigan gal.

I knew it would take practice, but what I was doing wasn't all that difficult and I couldn't even do it once without screwing up, let alone the thousands and thousands of times required for a scarf. In fact, my theory is "A scarf can *never* be too small."

I left the knitting place (or as I like to call it, the Frustration Emporium) a little tipsy, to say the least. I'm so paranoid about driving drunk, anyway. Years ago, after having a couple of drinks with dinner, I got stopped for not yielding to a pedestrian and the cop made me get out of the car for a sobriety test; I had to touch my nose and count backward in front of a senior citizens' home about a mile from my house. As I tried to avoid jail time, a collection of seniors gawked and the incessant mumbling really flirted with my concentration. Fortunately, I passed the balance test, counting drill and answered all of the officer's questions satisfactorily, thereby avoiding having to blow into any contraption that would dispense integers. I received a ticket only for my failure to yield. But it occurred to me that, like 99 percent of Americans, I had absolutely *no idea* if I was legally drunk. So the minute I got home I bought a Breathalyzer online for $89. Now I know—even before I blow into it—within one-tenth of a point where my body is on the alcohol blood-level percentage chart. Since I suspected I could very well be legally drunk, I didn't bother blowing into it; it would just make me even more paranoid on the ride home.

Had I been stopped, I would have undoubtedly been the first male in U.S. history to have a Breathalyzer in his glove compartment and get a DUI on his way back from a knitting class at seven-thirty at night.

But I made it home without incident.

And now I have a newfound respect for sweaters. I actually salute when I see one on a rack. But I don't like knitting. And honestly, I'm not crazy about knitters, either.

15

GRUDGING

My mother hasn't spoken to any of her brothers in at least thirty-five years. I don't even remember meeting two of the three. With a gun to my head I'd have a better chance of naming every National League Cy Young Award winner than my mother's siblings.

As I've said, my mother is the queen of grudges—against distant family, immediate family, the FedEx guy, the FedEx guy's family, Visa, the urologist who accidentally stepped on her foot. I'd always wondered if I had inherited some kind of genetic defect that encouraged grudges, because I could be just as obstinate as she. When I was in eleventh grade, Jeff Ulliano and Marty Kurtzman were supposed to call me to tell me where to meet them on a Thursday night of no significance. They said they forgot—although they hadn't forgotten to call Larry Bambus and Arnie Krever. That trivial oversight led me to break off the friendship with the entire group I had spent the better part of high school with, including countless Pink Floyd strobe-light shows at the local planetarium.

Because of my unbridled stubbornness, my senior year was the single worst year of my life. By twelfth grade, everyone was already in their cliques and had their circles of friends and it was hard to penetrate even the nerdiest of groups. I was the ultimate loner. I'd have been better off just transferring to another high school—at least then I'd be a fresh face who might arouse some curiosity. Instead, I took whatever social calendar scraps the dorks and geeks would dole out to me.

∘ ∘ ∘

A grudge is nothing more than stored hostility. Maybe my mother's resentful cravings had ignited her disease, just as my affinity for rapid aggression had undermined my body's defenses. I needed to find out if I was sentenced to a life of rancor, so I did some Googling and discovered that one of my mother's brothers, Lawrence, lived in Eugene, Oregon. A long drive, but far better than trekking to Maine or "somewhere in Wisconsin," which is where my mother's other brothers supposedly lived.

I hadn't seen Lawrence since I was five or six. I called him on the phone and lied. I told him that Nancy and I were going to be in Portland during Thanksgiving weekend visiting friends who had just had a baby, and we'd love to take him to dinner—if he was at all available or interested. He couldn't have been nicer and said that he and his wife (I had no idea he was even married) would love to see us. Maybe I wasn't saddled with the grudge gene. Maybe all this driving would be a complete waste of time.

He said he wasn't available on Thanksgiving, since they were "going down to the homeless shelter for the free meal." Was he really poor and reliant on soup kitchens for food? Or was he cheap? Or was it just a modest way of implying that he's going to be donating his time that day by helping others? Or was he making a joke at the expense of the homeless?

Much to ponder on the thirteen-hour drive to Eugene for a single meal.

On the way up, Nancy and I passed several almond farms.

"Where do almonds come from?" she asked.

"I have no idea."

"Me either."

"Do they grow in the dirt? Do they grow on trees? Do they come out of a snail's ass? It's really embarrassing that neither of us knows."

"I wish I had a BlackBerry. We could Google it."

"Where do blackberries come from?"

"Not sure."

"Little plants, I bet."

"Sounds right."

After I'd spent about three hours thumping the gas pedal, my sciatica—another souvenir from my 1982 street brawl—was sending shooting pains down my right leg. It was killing me to the point where I had to drive with my left foot, which Nancy would have flipped out about had I told her. Unfortunately, she couldn't drive, since we had forgotten to pack the yellow pages, so my left foot and I pressed on.

Since Nancy and I were both on strict Ayurvedic diets, we knew it would be challenging to find a place on the road for either of us to eat, let alone both of us. The freeway's domination of fast-food chains forced us to lower the bar. We chose Jack in the Box.

"I can eat chicken."

"So can I!"

"Black beans?"

"No. Corn?"

"Uh-uh."

"We'll just pick off the stuff we're not allowed to eat, then."

"Sure."

Nancy ordered some chicken fajita thing, since she was allowed—in fact, *encouraged!*—to eat spicy foods. I settled for the chicken sourdough sandwich—no sauce. We ate as I drove. However, as soon as I swallowed my first bite, something felt wrong. I slowly opened my sandwich to see what had provided the unexpected taste. I had just eaten a mouthful of bacon! Motherfuckers!!! I had given up bacon in 1979, six years before I'd stopped eating red meat. I was traumatized. (Incidentally, I hate it when people say, "Well, you eat chicken and fish, why not meat? That's really random of you." Oh yeah, well, you eat meat but I bet you don't eat dog and cat so shut up and come up with a better analogy!)

Even though we were at least fifteen minutes away from

Jack in the Box, I turned the car around and headed back to track down the manager. I needed to find out why there was bacon on my fucking chicken when it was never even mentioned on the menu.

I left Nancy in the car and burst into the Jack.

"Excuse me? Can I speak to a manager?"

"He's on break. I'm the assistant manager," said a bespectacled overweight guy in his sixties who seemed way too old to have his job, or any job for that matter.

"Um . . . yeah . . ." I held the remainder of my sandwich aloft. "I'd just like to know why there's bacon on my chicken sourdough sandwich!"

"Because there's supposed to be bacon on it, sir."

"Well, why wasn't it listed on the menu? Or why isn't it called a chicken AND BACON sourdough sandwich? Wouldn't that make sense to at least list the main ingredients?"

"You should have asked, sir."

So I was supposed to *ask* if there's bacon in everything? Is there bacon in the fries? Is there bacon in the pumpkin shake? Is there bacon in the Diet Pepsi? All this thinking about my mother and her brothers and grudges dredged up anger that even my Zoloft/Ayurvedic team were powerless against. I tried thinking about Bread of Shame but that, too, was useless at the moment.

"The sandwich you ordered is actually called 'The Sourdough Grilled Chicken *Club*,'" he continued.

"So?" I grew up eating "club" sandwiches and all it meant was that there was a third layer of bread between the other two slices. There was never any bacon on my club sandwiches. "Y'know what? I'll come back when the manager's here."

Then I slammed the remains of my sandwich down on the counter as if I were trying to bounce a basketball over a mountain and stormed out to fill in Nancy. If I had a can of spray paint I probably would've added the word "bacon" to the drive-thru menu on the way out.

"How'd it go?"

"Not good. He gave me this 'club-sandwich-means-it-has-bacon' bullshit."

"I think club *does* mean it has bacon."

"I don't think so. And on the way back from Oregon, I'm gonna stop and speak to the manager."

I suppose adding an extra grudge on the way to see if my grudges were inherited was poetic.

Ten hours later we checked into a local Eugene hotel, rested, changed and had sex, thanks to Nancy's being on vacation and my having lowered my dosage. Then I called my uncle Lawrence and told him we were on our way and he gave us an actual address.

We snaked our way along narrow roads and pulled up to a wood-stained farmhouse. Before I could even get out of the car there he was, waiting in the driveway. Lawrence was a large man, in the six-foot-two range with gray hair, thick glasses and a beard. He wore a blue-and-red flannel shirt, jeans and white Adidas sneakers, and despite being about thirty pounds over-weight and at least twenty years older than I am, he had a very bouncy, adolescent gait.

"You haven't changed a bit," he said drily as he extended his large, meaty hand.

"Neither have you." I smiled.

Nancy and I followed him inside as three yellow Labs greeted us. Then we met his wife, Sharon, who looked to be about five years older than Lawrence (although I knew so little about him, at the time I had no idea if he was even older or younger than my mother). The house was immaculate and much hipper than I'd expected for older people in Oregon. There were several fire-places, stainless steel appliances, a kidney-shaped couch and hardwood floors. Nancy and I could have lived in that house. Al-though she probably would have wanted all the butterflies taken off the walls. Actually, that's basically all there was on the walls. Framed butterflies. Dozens and dozens of framed butterflies.

"Whose butterflies?" I was perhaps the shrewdest conversation starter in all of the Pacific Northwest.

"They're Sharon's. She's been collecting them for years."

"Actually," said Sharon, who had a raspy Vanessa Redgravey voice, "some of them are moths."

"Moths! Wow!" Nancy exclaimed, pretending to be interested though I knew she was repulsed.

I wondered why people would want to trap these harmless creatures and stuff them into a picture frame. And how hard was it to catch a moth? Who was that supposed to impress? Just leave your front light on and grab a newspaper.

"So what brings you guys up here?" Sharon asked.

"Just visiting friends."

"Who just had a baby!" Nancy exclaimed, as we had rehearsed. If my uncle knew we had driven thirteen hours just to see if he was a bitter fuck, too, it would've really put a strain on the evening.

"So . . . I know that you and my mother haven't spoken in some time . . ."

"No, we haven't."

The only thing I knew about Lawrence was that he and his brother, Ted, had sent my mother that sympathy card when Andrew was born. But I didn't want to be angry at someone over something he mailed in 1963.

"Do you speak to your brothers regularly?"

"Yeah. It's been about twelve years since I spoke with Ted and sixteen years since I spoke with Bernie."

Either there was something to my grudge-gene theory or the meaning of "regularly" needed to be loosened.

The entire nature-nurture argument has always mystified me. If my mother and her family had a predisposition toward anger and ill will, was it learned or a preprogrammed mechanism that showed up at birth? And is it possible for nurture to change nature? The people at Pfizer think so. I hoped so.

Sharon put some nuts and cheese out and poured us each

wine. Unfortunately, it had sulfites. I guzzled it anyway. My uncle cut right to the chase.

"Your mother had a very tough life."

"I know."

"I mean even before the MS. She was seventeen years old and had to share a room with Ted and me. We're twelve years apart so I must've been five and Ted was seven or eight. It was hard for her."

How much could a seventeen-year-old girl and a five-year-old boy have in common, even if they are brother and sister? Their grudge could be just an excuse for permanent distance, which began emotionally and ended physically.

"Why is she mad at everyone?"

"I don't know. I haven't seen your mother in almost forty years."

"What about her other brothers?"

"You'd have to ask your mother, but I think part of it may have had to do with Bernie and Maureen naming their son Andrew."

Nancy sat in silence. Stunned. My mother's brother had intentionally named his only child after my dead brother? What sense did that make? Andrew wasn't even a family name. It had no significance. Except perhaps to torture my mother. That was really dicky of them. It's not like they had nineteen kids and were running out of names. Buttons were certainly being pushed. At the very least it was disrespectful.

"Why couldn't they have named him something else?"

"They liked the name Andrew," he said with a shrug.

"These almonds are good," interrupted Nancy.

"Yes, they're delicious," said Sharon.

"Where do they come from?"

"Our farm."

"No, I mean what part of your farm?"

"We also have a beef with your mother for financial reasons," Lawrence blurted. "When my mother, your grandmother, died, Rhoda was in charge of the estate."

"I barely remember that."

"Well," my uncle continued, "by the time your mother was through with all the paperwork and wheeling and dealing, the rest of us barely got anything."

This was a new one. My mother was a lot of things but she certainly wasn't a thief.

"I just don't believe that my mother would ever rip anyone off. Even a nickel."

"Well, we all think she did."

"Believe me, there was never even the slightest influx of money in our house."

"She claims that they didn't get much for the condo in Florida and that the lawyers were expensive."

That sounded logical.

"Did she offer you receipts?"

"Yeah, but who cares about receipts? Those are easy to forge."

So now my mother had a double major: stealing and forgery.

"Actually," he went on, "nobody even bothered to tell me that my mother had died until months later."

"You weren't in contact with her either?"

"No. I mean, I wouldn't have gone to the funeral anyway, but it still would've been nice to know."

"Why wouldn't you have gone to the funeral?"

"When my father died in 1979 I didn't go. Funerals are a waste of time. Anyway, when your grandmother—my mother— died, I was in no position to travel."

"That's when Lawrence was shot," said Sharon sadly.

"You were shot?!" Nancy and I asked in unison.

"Yeah. In 1985. I was living in East Flatbush running a stamp dealership out of my apartment. On the way home from the bank, a guy on a bicycle followed me and shot me three times in broad daylight just as I was getting into my elevator."

"He almost died."

"I still have one of the bullets in me somewhere."

"Are you okay now?"

"Yeah."

Two of the yellow Labs were jostling over which got to lick me.

"You know your grandmother—my mother—was allegedly involved with another man right after your grandfather died."

"I didn't know that. I barely knew her."

"She told me the guy took her for a lot of money."

"So maybe that's what happened to your inheritance? And it had nothing to do with my mother?"

"Your grandmother was addicted to barbiturates and amphetamines. Uppers and downers. Who knows what state she was in when she told me that?"

I had no inkling that my grandmother was a self-medicated pill junkie holed up in bed. And, if true, I wondered how much of an influence that was on my mother.

I knew that my grandfather wrote college textbooks but Lawrence told me he was also a ghostwriter.

"He actually ghostwrote a book called *How to Control Your Blood Pressure* by a guy named Dr. Alexander Pomerantz. I think it was an Ace Books paperback."

The fact that my late grandfather had ghostwritten a book for a doctor on blood pressure was alone worth the drive to Oregon.

"Did your mother ever tell you about *Dennis the Dizzy Dinosaur?*"

"No."

"It was a children's book she wrote. It was probably in the late fifties. Your father illustrated it. They sent it to some publishers and the response was that dinosaurs were too scary for kids. Two months later, Sinclair Oil unveiled a dinosaur as their mascot and kids loved it."

"How was the book?"

"I have to say I really liked it."

We then went out to a really nice restaurant and spoke about Sharon's kids, grandkids, writing, computers and television shows. They were both really interesting people who, had they

lived a little closer to us, we would have loved to see on a regular basis. And my uncle was a very cool, nice, smart guy—even
before he insisted on picking up the check. I felt kind of bad for
lying about the reason for our visit, but it seemed like a safe lie.
Who would drive twenty-six hours round-trip just to see why
his mother's siblings didn't speak to one another? At last now I
had a little bit of closure. My mother had a tough life, continues
to have a tough life, and grudges never make things any easier.

On the drive home, I didn't stop at Jack in the Box.

16

REIKI-ING

I had learned a valuable lesson from our trip to Oregon. Let things go immediately or they can fester forever. The thirteen-hour drive back to Los Angeles was one of the most tranquil days I'd ever experienced, and certainly the mellowest I'd ever been in a car.

In the meantime, for my birthday Nancy had bought me a series of private yoga classes at our house. Although my previous experience nearly ripped my hip out of my pelvis and set me back enough money to buy 1,700 yellowtail handrolls, I was healed and willing to give yoga a second chance. It's always worked for Nancy, who assured me that the instructor was aware of my past troubles and would keep a close eye on me. After the first at-home, I felt amazing. The Zoloft, Ayurvedic diet, Tai Chi and yoga were working in synergy.

Even Nancy agreed that I could soon drop myself down to 50 mg.

While cleaning out my car, I unearthed a glossy pamphlet for something called "Reiki by Sandi" that I'd found on a bulletin board in a Jamba Juice—where, incidentally, I am no longer allowed to frequent; the drinks are too cold and the bulk of the ingredients aren't Ayurveda-friendly.

According to the literature, Reiki (pronounced "ray-key") "releases stress, increases tranquillity, accelerates the body's ability to heal physical ailments" and "medical studies have shown that treatment results in a significant reduction in anxiety." This would allegedly be accomplished by the moving around of energy, and, I'd assumed, some words of wisdom thrown my way. Like Ayurveda, Reiki's been around for over

5,000 years. Unlike with Ayurveda, one is fully clothed for the procedure. Again, I was psyched to try something new.

When I called the number on the pamphlet I was saddened to learn that it had been disconnected. Apparently, the three-color printing had eaten away at Sandi's Reiki profits and she had to close up shop.

As I searched through phone books and the Internet for another Reiki master, I stumbled upon an alternative solution to alternative medicine. Distance Reiki. It would cost a mere $10 for a ten-minute session and I wouldn't have to drive anywhere. Plus, there were over 800,000 Google matches, so it had to be legit. I paid through PayPal and made an appointment via e-mail. The following is my entire correspondence with "Matrika."

12/14 7:14 PM
Hi Brian,
Looks like you've paid for a short, individual Reiki session. When you request an individual session like this, I try to make it available at a time that is best for you so long as I can fit it into my relatively flexible schedule. So here are my questions for you: do you have any specific health concerns you're interested to have me focus on, or would you simply like a general healing? In the latter case, I often intuit things that ought to be focused on anyway, but I'd like to first address things according to your preference. Second, is there a specific time and day when you would like to have this session, or would you like me to simply do this at my earliest convenience? Usually people who request a specific time do so in order to focus themselves on the sessions. Please let me know what you'd like.
Sincerely,
Matrika

12/15 12:55 PM
i'd love a general healing. if you have any time tomorrow (friday) that would be great and i could rearrange my schedule accordingly.
best,
brian

12/16 12:52 PM

Brian, I'm going to provide a Reiki session for you at 4:00 EST today (in 10 minutes). Sorry for the short notice. I will provide another session for you at another time if you're unable to focus in on this one.
Matrika

12/16 1:16 PM

sorry. can't do it then. i need a little more notice than that.

Eight minutes notice! What the hell is that? And why was he/she assuming I'm always online (even though I am always online)? Attempting to schedule this ten-minute session was starting to drain me.

12/16 1:24 PM

I figured you would need more notice. I had forgotten to schedule something earlier, but I also wanted to provide a session today since you asked for one. That's why I'm happy to also schedule something for another day. You let me know what day. I had a perception during the session. This may have just been coming to MY mind, but often in a session like this, I find I'm able to perceive something about the other person. Seems to me you've got a lot of things running through your head—not just the thoughts that most people have, but almost like actual voices saying specific things. This could just be ideas coming to you or it could be some form of ESP, whether consciously used or not. Are you at all aware of having these types of experiences?
Matrika.

12/16 2:49 PM

i'm not all that aware of the voices. i'm around until 4:15 PST if you have any time. if not, sometime early saturday would be good . . . does this take place over the phone (which i had assumed) or strictly via e-mail?
best,
brian

12/17 9:59 AM
Brian, via e-mail. It is a distance Reiki session. The only reason for contact is to set up a time in case you want to be concentrating on the session. That's not even critical, but some people like to do it to see what
they can perceive during the session. It's 10:00 a.m. your time right
now and I just got your message about doing it this morning. I'm probably heading out for a little bit. If you'd like to arrange for something
today, please make it later this afternoon or evening so I'll have time to
see your message and confirm the time with you.
Sincerely,
Matrika.

*I was getting pissed. This shouldn't have been this much of a hassle
for ten minutes of her time over the Internet. (Nancy insisted Matrika
was female because the name ends in an a.)*

12/17 10:20 AM
how about 1 o'clock pacific time, 4 o'clock your time?
brian

*Okay . . . I'd been sitting around, staring at my in-box for six
hours, which to me was not a "little bit." I felt like a moron waiting
for someone to answer an e-mail. Plus, I had a Christmas party that
I didn't want to go to but had to and it was football season and I
knew they wouldn't have the game on there and I'd be lucky if there
was a morsel of anything Ayurvedic I could eat. I couldn't believe my
day revolved around the writing whims of some irresponsible Reiki
lady—especially after I'd PAID her $10 to "work" with me. For ten
fucking minutes! That's $60 an hour! I wrote another e-mail, this
time using CAPS to emphasize my displeasure.*

12/17 6:02 PM
okay . . . please tell me WHEN YOU CAN DO THIS SESSION and i'll
make it a point to be around. i didn't think it would drag on like this for
a ten-minute session.
brian

12/18 7:56 PM

Hi Brian,

I do apologize for the drag-out. Again, this is why I had that first session anyway, to sort of double up on the actual Reiki time since I missed you on Friday. Anyway, got caught up in family things on Saturday. I am available most of the day on Monday. I will plan NOON YOUR TIME on Monday unless you drop me a line telling me another time. This way something is definitely scheduled but you can still arrange it as you like if you prefer something different.

Sincerely,

Matrika.

12/18 8:26 PM

noon (pacific time) on monday sounds great! i'll be online.

best,

Brian

12/19 11:57 AM

Hi Brian,

Just a quick note to say that I'm about to begin your session.

Matrika.

Good! She's starting on time. I've rearranged my entire day over this ten-minute burst of insanity.

12/19 11:58 AM

great! i'm here.

Brian

12/19 1:04 PM

should i be doing anything?

So I sat for over an hour and she didn't write me back a fucking word. I wondered if I just had way too many things wrong with me for her to type—perhaps Matrika was an awful typist who only pecked with her index fingers. Waiting to heal is one thing but wait-

ing for someone to answer an e-mail sucks. Bread of Shame! Bread
of Shame!

   An hour later I had a feeling this was all a scam.

   Another two hours later—nearly four full hours since she was about
to "begin our session"—I still hadn't heard from Matrika. I'm a god-
damned sap! I should've let things go but I couldn't. Another grudge
had sprouted. Despite my spending thousands of dollars on trying to
calm down, this $10 I was taken for was gnawing at me. The odd
thing is that the big things in life I can handle better than most peo-
ple—deaths, illness, losing a job—because I know there's nothing I can
do about them. It's the little things that get me riled up because I un-
duly believe that I can change and affect the outcome. Which I know
isn't practical because I usually can't. Damn, I could've used that
extra 50 mg boost.

   12/19 3:49 PM
   i'm contesting the charges with pay pal, scam artist!!!

Two hours later I checked my PayPal account. The $10 had
been transferred back to me by a guy named Pete with a hot-
mail address. Nancy was wrong.

I was still determined to do Reiki, but this time the traditional
way. I Googled some more and found a Reiki woman in
Tarzana. I called for an appointment and told her about my desire to calm down.

   "Oh, you're gonna love this, then. It's great for getting rid of
stress."

   It's also great for adding stress if the concept is poorly com-
municated to you and you have a PayPal account.

   "Good. Should I bring anything?"

   "Just some comfortable clothes. Oh, and you'll be coming to
my home office. Is that all right?"

   "Sure. Fine."

   I showed up in my sweats at über-suburbia. Predictably, I
was forty minutes early and decided I didn't want to be seen

lurking in front of her house. There was a school and play-ground a block away and I didn't want anyone thinking I was a perv. It's a similar feeling to the paranoia I experience when I walk into a store with something I already own and think they'll arrest me for shoplifting. That's why I often wave the previously purchased product in the air when I enter such a business, in hopes that their video surveillance cameras will verify proof of my ownership.

So, instead of being mistaken for a child molester, I'd try to be productive. I decided to get my car washed. While strangers with the keys to my vehicle were allegedly vacuuming and cleaning it, I would kill some time in the "gift shop." Now, unless one collects things that hang from a rearview mirror or yearns for breath mints, there wasn't really much to buy. Then I saw something that would seemingly occupy me for a while. It was a large rotating Lucite tower filled with individual let-ters in separate compartments that could be used to build a customized bracelet. I was excited. I'd make one for Nancy that said something stupid on it. However, I soon noticed that it would be a nearly impossible task.

"Um . . . excuse me . . . but there are no a's . . . do you have any more a's? Or e's or b's, actually," I said as I spun the tower around, searching frantically for vowels.

"Sorry," the cashier politely responded. "No a's."

I couldn't even spell "frustration." Either get rid of the dis-play or replenish the letters! Why does shit like that infuriate me? Is it the bad business sense of the owners? Is it the general apathy of people? Or is it my disappointment in myself be-cause I really don't buy Nancy enough presents and have to rely on a car wash for my holiday shopping? I felt like knocking over the entire display by dragging my forearm across it as if angrily clearing a restaurant table. Then maybe my aggression would randomly spell some words on the sticky car wash gift shop floor. Although the preponderance of x's and z's made that unlikely.

◦ ◦ ◦

I entered an old Spanish-style home and was greeted by my Reiki-ist. Claire was in her late twenties, had curly red hair and a giant hoop through her pierced nose. Every time I looked at Claire's nose ring, it just reminded me how dry my nose currently was. In the haste to get out of my house, I'd forgotten to Q-tip my baby rash ointment up each nostril. And the dry Santa Ana winds were now punishing my septum for the forgetfulness.

There was incense burning, wind chimes chiming, candles flickering; the calmness seemed pompous.

"Do you need to use the bathroom?"

I didn't but maybe she'd have some Vaseline or hair conditioner I could shove up my nostrils for some relief. Some Chap-Stick might even do the trick.

"Yes, please."

I went into the bathroom but there wasn't much of anything, except soap. I needed some shaving cream, sunscreen, anything that would be even minutely moister than my nostrils. I would've even considered toothpaste; however, this was a minimalist guest bathroom and I believe there's no reason for my nose to ever smell better than my mouth. I should have just asked if she had some Vaseline-like substance in another bathroom. Surely someone with a pierced nostril would understand dry nose issues. I'm sure that probably-not-gold-plated hoop dangling above her upper lip has irritated the surrounding skin at least once. Maybe some water would do for me in the meantime. But what if that just dried me out more? I had to take the chance. I stuck my nose in the sink and tried to get the faucet directly above my left nostril, in hopes of flooding the dryness out. Unfortunately, all I did was get several gallons of water all over my sweatshirt and make my nose drippy and dry.

"Are you okay in there?" Claire asked.

"Yeah . . . just washing my face!"

"All right. Let me know if you need anything."

"Um . . . I could use a sweatshirt . . . if you have an extra one . . . I think I got mine wet."

She must've wondered what the hell I was doing in there.
"I may have an oversize one that'll fit."

"Okay. Thanks!"

Four minutes later my nose was still dry and I was lying flat on my stomach on a massage table while wearing a gray Minnie Mouse sweatshirt that belonged to Claire's mother. I'm an idiot.

"I don't remember what you told me on the phone. Have you ever had Reiki before?"

Dammit, was my nose dry!

"Technically no. I tried Distance Reiki once but it didn't work out."

"Well, this will."

Claire rubbed her hands together furiously, as if she were trying to start a fire, then placed them very, very lightly on the back of my head. After a minute or two, her hands inched down toward my neck for another couple of minutes, then on to my upper back, mid-back, hamstrings . . . you get the idea.

Exactly what was happening to me, I didn't know. Claire explained that, unlike spiritual healing, where the healer sends out the energy, in Reiki it is the recipient who draws the necessary energy from the person touching them. So instead of her hands sucking out my bad energy, the burden was on me to take good energy out of her. Unfortunately, I had no idea how to steal somebody's energy. Did I have to trick it into coming near the surface of Claire's skin so I could just drag it into my pores? And even if I was adept at taking energy, what if I took the bad kind by mistake? Or what if this was another scam and she was sucking all the good energy out of me to sell to someone else? Bottom line: despite all the flowery language, as I lay there it just felt like Claire was a really lazy person who was supposed to massage me but didn't feel like it.

Halfway through our session, I flipped over onto my back and she started touching the front half of me. Shit, was my nose dry! I should have just asked her for some cream. Any kind of cream! Every woman has cream in her pocketbook, let alone her home.

Why didn't I ask for some cream?! Bread of Shame! Bread of Shame! My dried-out nostrils would inevitably teach me some sort of important life lesson. I just didn't know what yet.

All of a sudden there was a lot of commotion. At first I thought Claire was being robbed—but not of her energy, of more tangible items, like a laptop. Then I realized it was her roommate coming home. With a dog. A very frisky dog. A very frisky dog that kept scurrying back and forth down the hardwood hallway with his very long nails. We were almost done. Why couldn't the roommate have come home just fifteen minutes later? I'm sure her car could've used a wash—unless she, too, was frustrated at the lack of popular consonants with which to build a bracelet. Throughout the disturbance, Claire was oblivious and kept touching me. She was now down to my belly button. I had forgotten to tell her that I can't tolerate my belly button being touched. It feels like a dead spot on my body, kind of like some dead nerves on the side of my neck that I have to avoid while shaving. No one gets to touch my belly button! Not even Nancy. I should have just put scaffolding over it or glued a dime onto it for protection. But neither of us had said a word for the past thirty-five minutes and I didn't want to break the silence. I'd let the scampering dog do that.

What was the dog running from anyway? He had just come from outside so he should be zonked out on a fluffy dog pillow somewhere. And why not clip the dog's nails? Or take him somewhere to get them clipped if you're too nervous that you're going to hit a blood vessel doing it yourself? The noise was starting to grate on me. Now I fully understood the term "home office."

Rip. Rip. Rip. Now what? Her roommate was ripping up junk mail or the statements for bills that had just been paid. Or just being obnoxious. Or all three of those things. Scamper, scamper, scamper. Rip, rip, rip. At least invest in a shredder! In comparison, the motorized mincing would be soothing, which ripping never is. Unless one is the person doing the ripping.

Miraculously the ripping and scampering simultaneously stopped and peace was restored. Until three seconds later when I was startled by some loud grinding. Jesus Christ! Blender drinks! Couldn't this wait three more minutes? Does anyone REALLY need a frozen margarita at one in the afternoon? As the last of the ice cubes were crushed by the whirring metal blades, Claire removed her hands from me. My time was up.

"How do you feel?"

I had hoped that all the noises hadn't distracted me from sucking out the maximum of Claire's positive energy.

"Relaxed, I guess."

I did feel relaxed; however, I had been lying down for the past fifty minutes. If Nancy had blown on my toes for an hour, I'm not sure the results would've been any different.

"Now, take your time getting off the table. And you might experience an even deeper sense of relaxation tomorrow."

"Okay. Did you find anything odd inside me during the session?"

"Actually, when I put my hands over your heart chakra, I got a little frightened at first."

"Really?"

"I think there's a problem with acceptance in your heart."

What?! My heart accepts stuff! I got married, I have friends, I really get along with the mailman. . . . But if she's right, maybe this "acceptance" issue comes back to religion and that whole Jewish conundrum with my rabbi. And how fate had treated my mother. I wondered if everything came back to God.

"And anger. There's anger in your heart, too."

Duh.

Now, here's the weird thing. While I was still in the privacy of her spare-bedroom/massage table/home-office room with the door shut, I asked her if her dog had beagle and dachshund in it.

"Oh my God! It's a beagle-dachshund mix! How did you know?"

"I don't know."

I really didn't know how I knew. I'm terrible at guessing

stuff. I can't even get *one* lottery number right. Maybe all of her touching had released something in me that allowed me to see through walls, or at least guess dog breeds based on how their paws sounded on hardwood. Or maybe Matrika/Reiki Pete was onto something when he said I had actual voices running through my head that could be some form of ESP. Maybe I was a dick for getting my money back from PayPal.

On the way home I stopped for gas. As soon as I got out to start pumping, I noticed that I was getting a few stares. At first I thought that word had spread quickly about my dog breed predicting abilities. Then I looked down and realized I was still wearing a snug Minnie Mouse sweatshirt.

I felt calm enough to not take my Zoloft that afternoon. It was the first time I had ever intentionally skipped a day. I guess I was just getting sick of all the excuses and wanted desperately to taper down to 50 mg. The remainder of the evening and the following day I was extremely light-headed and dizzy. Was it the aftermath of the Reiki? Was it because I had neglected my magic pill the previous day? Was it the Santa Ana winds again? Or, when I smashed up my weekly Ayurvedic coconut with a hammer in my driveway, had I inadvertently eaten some asphalt? In any event, I didn't feel well. I probably should've taken my pill.

The next week, Claire called to see if I wanted to set up another appointment. I decided not to. Those frenetic scraping dog claws combined with the potential of her roommate getting involved with an even more annoying hobby, like indoor bowling, didn't make me want to shell out another $60. Besides, Nancy's energy was just as good as hers. From then on I'd just suck some out of her while we were spooning. However, upon learning of my plan, Nancy preferred that I leave her good energy alone—although I had dibs on the bad stuff.

17

PETTING

"He seems nice. Sure."

Nancy and I had just adopted a dog from a shelter. We'd been looking for months but could never agree on one. She wanted something she could bring to work inside her pocketbook and I wanted to retain my heterosexuality.

We chose Toto, as he was then called, because of his composure. Although chaos reigned as he was engulfed by a slew of aggressively barking canines and screaming kids with argumentative parents, our soon-to-be pet remained unflappable. He was the calmest dog I had ever seen—so calm, in fact, that I wondered if he was medicated. It was hard to believe he was just three months old. If he was this composed as a puppy, it boded well for his future demeanor. And perhaps mine.

Studies have shown that pet owners live longer. Prisoners and hospital patients have lowered their blood pressure, cholesterol and triglyceride levels in the company of animals; heart attack victims have a better survival rate; Alzheimer's patients have a decrease in mood disorders; seizure sufferers report that their dogs can sense the onset of a convulsion before they can. And a service dog can prevent a Parkinson's patient from falling by touching his owner's feet when they're frozen in place. If dogs could do all that, then helping me slow down seemed a reasonable expectation.

Although my family always had dogs while I was growing up, they were as unsocialized and volatile as the human inhabitants who fed them. Besides almost killing that cable guy, Rufus had nearly come to blows with many of our neighbors. Whenever a friend came over, Wally had to be held and then dragged into a distant area of the house to ensure the friend's safety. Sydney's personality was as unpredictable as his sudden death from a staph infection. Were the dogs crazy or did we make them crazy? Nature or nurture? Regardless, I was elated to have my first pet that probably wouldn't hurt anyone.

The name had to go. First of all, he looked nothing like Toto. Dorothy's Toto was a cairn terrier and our new dog was an Irish terrier–border terrier mix whose rumpled, scraggly hair always gave the appearance that he had just woken up. (He also looks nothing like Benji, so please stop saying that when you see me walking him. I'm serious. IMDb "Benji" and I'm sure you'll agree. I'm considering downloading a picture of Benji and keeping it in my wallet so when strangers definitively say, "Hey, it's Benji!" I can pull out the evidence and retort, "No, it's *not*. My dog is tall, angular and wirehaired while Benji is short, squat and fluffy and has larger, floppy ears. In fact, my mutt looks very much like a live-action version of the tramp from *Lady and the Tramp* and nobody would compare the tramp to Benji. Now go take a class in visual memorization!") In any event, I would *not* be saying the word "Toto" aloud in my home, unless I was asked who sang that shitty song "Rosanna." Despite his gentle manner, for some reason Nancy and I wound up naming him after Kenyon Martin, one of the fiercest, most combustible players in the NBA.

Although we'd been living in the same house for five years, since we drove everywhere, we didn't really know any of our neighbors, but this didn't stop me from holding phantom grudges against them based on the subtleties of facial expressions I witnessed from my car. The shaved-headed motherfucker was a conceited asshole; the pretty lady with the ugly attitude was a bitch; the guy with the Mercedes jeep was a Nazi. However, walking Kenyon up and down the block three or four times a day forced me into face-to-face encounters with people whom I'd never seen without a car window separating us. It turned out the shaved-headed motherfucker was a gregarious landscape artist and as die-hard a basketball fan as I was; the pretty lady with the ugly attitude owned a goat milk ice cream company and did volunteer environmental work; and the guy with the Mercedes Nazi jeep was a famous movie poster designer who gave us a $100 bottle of wine for the holidays. All of my pent-up animosity was fictitious and had no grounding in reality. One might think that any dog would have united me with our neighbors; however, there are plenty of people who walk dogs on our street that nobody wants to talk to. A lot of it inevitably has to do with Kenyon's personality.

Unlike me, Kenyon accepted things for what they were. Since we crate-trained him, at the end of each day we'd usher him into a cage. Naturally, he would have preferred sleeping in our bed or even on the floor next to the window, but he entered without protest. When walking on a leash and spotting another dog, he'd get excited but never attempt to pull. He knew we'd get there eventually. And he was even judicious when eating. I'd been accustomed to seeing a dog attack food, much as I did, as if every meal were a race. Kenyon took his time and delicately savored each bite, rarely finishing what was in his bowl. Even though he'd only been on the planet for thirteen weeks, he quickly became my role model.

Like the dogs that can sense seizures, Kenyon was magically able to anticipate my moods and actions. On our first drive alone together, he sat perched in the passenger seat and, without the added height of Nancy's lap, was way too small to actually see anything over the window or dashboard. Within five minutes, a car cut in front of me without signaling. Before I could even react to the other driver, the mutt scratched me with his tiny paw, as if he were requesting my composure. I had no choice but to accede to his wish. I didn't want to upset him. Unlike my laminated cards, mantras and pills, Kenyon would be affected by my actions. Not that Nancy wasn't, but she had the power to get out of the car at a red light and walk away. Kenyon was stuck with me.

I was remarkably calmer whenever Kenyon was by my

side—which became pretty much all the time. Within a week I had folded up the crate and he was sleeping in bed with us. The rhythmic beating of his tiny terrier heart induced deeper and more restful nights. If I couldn't get off the Zoloft with the help of his wirehaired presence, I'd never be able to. I was in love. And so was Nancy. The combination of Ayurveda, Kenyon and the strong possibility of her show ending finally started to de-stress her. The cumulative amounts of anxiety in our house reached their lowest levels since we'd moved in.

I developed a new mantra that helped me not to overreact: "What Would Kenyon Do?" Yeah, it sounds pretty lame but it's a great litmus test. When I got angry because a business call wasn't returned, I'd think aloud, "What Would Kenyon Do?" Easy. He'd lie in the sun and shut his eyes. When a cell phone went off in the movie theater, I'd wonder, "What Would Kenyon Do?" Simple. He'd listen to the semi-melodic tone and flash his pointy smile. When I was about to yell at someone who'd stolen the parking spot I'd been waiting for, I'd ponder, "What Would Kenyon Do?" He'd wag his tail at the people in the car. (Which I pretend to do but don't actually wiggle my ass.)

I never felt better in my life. I was finally able to anticipate the day I'd have the following conversation with Dr. Tamm.

"Hi, I feel fantastic."

"So you're ready?"

"Absolutely!"

"Good. You'll go down to 50 mg for a couple of weeks and, if all goes well, drop down to one pill every other day and then cut out the Zoloft completely."

I hoped never to enter my pharmacy again unless I was looking for batteries or sunscreen.

The following morning, the phone rang and derailed my fantasy. It was my sister calling from Florida. My father was in the emergency room. My only surprise was that it hadn't happened sooner. Rather than my mother being in an assisted-living facility or nursing home, my father had the unenviable job of lifting her up with his seventy-three-year-old back and transferring her broken body to the commode—every hour and a half. Every day. After all the constant awkward lifting, my father's back went out. Now they were both immobile and Debbie had too much on her plate.

I needed to fly down to Sarasota to run errands for my father and help out my mother. Unfortunately, that meant traveling without Kenyon. Despite his mere twenty-one pounds, his giraffelike legs were too tall for him to fit under the seat of an airplane. And he wasn't going cargo. He's an animal, not a piece of luggage.

We reluctantly dropped Kenyon off at a friend's house. Then, on the way to the airport, I wanted to go back and pick him up, eat the plane tickets and drive cross-country to Florida with Nancy and him. But she didn't want to be in a car with me unnecessarily for six days. I would have to do without my wiry mentor for a while. Fortunately, I had a backup plan. And, where I was going, I'd need one.

18

ERASING

The same day I booked our flights to Florida, I had a StressEraser FedExed. It was a $399 silver rectangle about the size of a deck of cards. Nancy instantly called it the Money-Eraser.

Yes, it may appear that I'm wasting my money. I'm certainly not rich. However, (a) the StressEraser came with a sixty-day money-back guarantee and (b) for me there's no such thing as wasting money if it's going toward my health. Adopting a star in the sky for $54—*that's* wasting money! Buying an expensive bar of soap—*that's* wasting money! Purchasing anything at the Sharper Image except for one of those Touchless Trashcans—*that's* wasting money!

Besides, I'm a minimalist. I don't have a lot of things. When I buy a shirt, I give one to Goodwill. When I buy a pair of sneakers, I get rid of a pair. I have enough clutter in my brain, I don't need it in my house.

My brother is the complete opposite. Mark attaches sentimental value to everything, and not just because he makes a living playing oldies. When my parents moved to Florida, he drove eleven and a half hours from Dayton, Ohio, to Long Island to pick up the shutters from our childhood home. He then made a *second trip* back to pick up the front door to our former residence after craftily negotiating a "fair price" with the new owners of $500, which didn't include the replacement door they demanded.

Mark has a one-car garage in a city that can have some pretty tough winters. Subsequently, one would think that a home owner would keep the car that he *drives to work every day* inside the confines of that lone warm garage stall. But my brother has other priorities. When he graduated from college in the late '70s our grandparents bought him a Toyota Celica as a gift. Although he hasn't been able to start its engine in well over two decades, the Celica sits comfortably in the garage while his functioning car lies in the cold and rusts.

It was while looking for parts for the ancient Celica on eBay that Mark came across a blue 1965 Nova, which happened to be the car my grandparents had driven from Brooklyn to Long Island like clockwork every Saturday morning when we were kids. They would arrive at ten o'clock sharp with toys and a large tub of butter cookies (non-Ayurvedic) that my grandmother had baked. They spoiled the hell out of us. So my brother promptly bid $3,700 on that Nova, then paid a friend another $400 to drive down to Kentucky and back to Dayton to transport it back. But wait. There's more. A week after purchasing *that* Nova, he was back surfing eBay when he came across . . . *another* blue '65 Nova! But this one had lower miles and was in better shape. So another $4,500 later, he had his fourth car, and his third that will never leave his driveway. And more debt on his menagerie of credit cards. When I questioned him as to why he needs two blue Novas that will get eaten alive by Dayton's winters and that he'll never use, he replied: "It's like Santa's sleigh. I look at that car and I'm eight years old again and Mom's healthy and doesn't have multiple sclerosis . . ." I know it's convenient and on-the-nose, but he really said that.

In the few days after I bought our plane tickets, my father's back had improved and he'd returned home. In the meantime, my mother had been in and out of the hospital again, this time with congestive heart failure. But after she was discharged, she was still unable to get to her commode an arm's length away without a transfer from my father, whose balky back couldn't yet accommodate her weight. Even under these dire circumstances, professional help was out of the question. Because that never worked out. Because my mother doesn't like anybody. And people in the medical field don't like her much, either.

While visiting, I planned to finally tell my mother that I was on Zoloft, hoping I could convince her to try some, too. With any luck she would realize there was nothing to be ashamed or embarrassed about. Without luck, she would think I was weak for being "healthy" and relying on pills as a crutch.

The StressEraser would be indispensable.

Our trip got off to an auspicious start at airport security. My bags were searched and I didn't travel like a typical passenger. Especially now.

"Excuse me, sir," said the tubby, armed guy. "What's that jar with the yellow stuff?"

"Ghee."

"Ghee?"

"It's Indian clarified butter."

"Why are you traveling with butter, sir?"

"My Ayurvedist made me."

"Ayurvedist?"

"It's a health thing."

He picked up my jar of herbs.

"Are these drugs?"

"No. They're herbs. Which are supposed to relax me." I could have used some then. Our flight was boarding in twenty minutes.

"Is this pot?"

"No!" I said a little too defensively. Why would anyone carry pot around in a big glass jar? "I mix it with my tea in the morning . . . and after lunch. And that clear jar in your other hand is aloe vera juice."

"I'm gonna have to ask you to go wait over there while I call my supervisor."

Bread of Shame! Bread of Shame! This will teach me patience, I thought to myself as Nancy was told to continue toward the gate.

It took me fifteen minutes to explain that my collection of Mason jars had nothing to do with building a nuclear warhead. The pieces started to fall into place for airport security when they questioned my little silver machine.

"Is that the new iPod?"

"No. It's a StressEraser."

"A *what?*"

"It's supposed to manage stress."

"How?"

"I have no idea. I'm gonna read the manual on the plane," I said, more nervous than I should have been. After waving his magic beeping stick across my body several more times and subconsciously realizing that no blond Jews have ever blown up a plane, the supervisor allowed me to catch up to Nancy at the gate.

I sat in my assigned window seat and attacked the manual.

The StressEraser would allegedly help to erase stress in three stages:

- Learning to calm your mind
- Learning to relax your body
- Learning to quiet your emotions

And, the StressEraser is intended to be used for:

- Relaxation
- Relaxation training
- Stress reduction

They really knew how to eat up space.

It was pretty simple to figure out. Basically, it's a pocket-size video game for breathing. You're supposed to stick an index finger into the StressEraser's sensor, which subsequently monitors pulse rate. Whenever a breath is taken, a square or series of squares appears along the bottom of the screen. A single square or two squares side by side results in zero points; two squares stacked vertically on top of each other add a half point; three squares stacked vertically add a full point—all of which registers in the upper left-hand corner of the device. According to the manual, "If you want to feel emotional relief, it's important to accumulate at least thirty points each session." Fifty or more points before sleep is also a good idea. Or they even recommend getting 100 points a day over a two-month period. Another good idea? Not buying the StressEraser.

As I breathed deeply with my finger attached to the small overpriced piece of metal, I felt a tap on my shoulder.

"Excuse me, sir." It was a middle-aged flight attendant with a red bow on her head.

"Yes?"

"You need to put away all electronic devices."

"But it's only a StressEraser and we're still on the runway."

"Please put it away until after takeoff. Or I'll have to confiscate it."

You'll get my StressEraser when you pry it from my cold, dead hands! I wanted to say.

"Sure. Sorry."

Once we were in the air, it was pretty simple to figure out the StressEraser and I was pretty disappointed. The gist of it: *Slow down my breathing.* I learned that during the first thirty seconds of my first yoga class. I didn't need to lug around a little silver box packed in way too much Styrofoam to realize it. I contemplated betting the elderly man on my left to see who could get the higher score, but I didn't even want to look at the StressEraser anymore. It disgusted me. Even the manual was filled with nonsense. "A common technique to deal with worry is to take a worry break." No wonder that, according to page 30 in booklet number 2, ". . . the FDA has not approved the StressEraser for the treatment of any condition." Because it's useless. I missed Kenyon.

o o o

I knew this trip would be different. First of all, Debbie had warned me how bad things were at home and suggested that Nancy and I stay in a hotel. I had never stayed in a hotel before when visiting my parents, although I had threatened to do so on numerous occasions. They had a decent-sized guest room and, despite the bedlam, there was no reason to Red-Roof-Inn it.

Second, my sister told me that my father would not be picking me up at the airport. When my parents lived on Long Island I was never picked up, since my father feared highway driving and it was nearly impossible to get to JFK via side streets. Now that they lived five minutes from an airport that was accessible by local roads, he was always there to get me. But not this time. He couldn't leave my mother alone for more than ten minutes. For the past few years it had been an hour. Now he was practically tethered to the house. I called the motel and booked a room.

DAY ONE

We took a taxi to my parents' house so we could pick up their extra car—which my mother had insisted on having in case of emergency. My father greeted us at the door. He had put on even more weight and now had the stomach of a fat white man and the ass of a fat black woman. His lone remaining joy in life was eating Breyers straight out of the half-gallon container. At this point, the only question was how much weight he would add to his frame in between my visits. I would have definitely lost to him in an ice cream eating contest; it appeared as if he had been training hard.

He was usually in a jovial mood when he had visitors, perhaps because they diluted my mother's presence. But this time there was nothing in his eyes but despair.

"Do you want to see your mother?"

"Sure. If she's ready."

"Let me go and check."

Five minutes later, after hearing a lot of bickering behind

closed doors, Nancy and I were allowed to enter her bedroom.

My mother's legs were swollen like an elephant's. Debbie had warned us about this. Fluids from her congestive heart failure had traveled into her calves. The next (and final) stop would be her lungs. Despite her mangled body, her skin remained in pristine condition. She still had the face and hands of a thirty-five-year-old, the lone perk from sitting in a dark room for three decades.

"Hello. How was your flight?"

"Fine."

After a brief respite, she went on the warpath.

"Where is the shit?"

"Huh?"

"Your fa-ther."

She's calling my father a shit ten seconds after seeing us? Nancy already looked uncomfortable. I simply ignored my mother.

"Look at this!" she ranted, pointing to her water glass, which was three-quarters full. "This is all I have to drink for the entire day!"

"I don't understand. You're only allowed one glass of water a day?"

"No! Your fa-ther ne-ver comes by to re-fill it!"

Bullshit! My mother has a series of plastic buzzers all over her bedroom and bathroom which she presses liberally to summon my dad, who races in each time as if he's a firefighter. I'd be shocked if during any twenty-four-hour period, she didn't see him for an hour. Sometimes she buzzes him in from his bedroom in the middle of the night simply to adjust the temperature a few degrees for her fickle inner thermostat. It's hard to evaluate someone's internal pain, but it couldn't have been much worse than the pain she inflicted on my father.

"*I* can get you some water, Mom."

"I don't ne-ed any wat-er right now! I will ne-ed some lat-er!"

"Well, I'm sure Dad will bring you some when you're ready."

"He's too busy look-ing in-to the lake!"

"What?"

"This morn-ing he was mar-vel-ing at a bird that had swooped down in-to the lake and *caught a fish*!"

Actually, that sounded pretty cool. So you're upset because he's not focused on you every waking second? I didn't know if my mother was getting worse, I was getting better, or both.

"And your sister just bought a king-size bed for Michelle!" she roared. Yelling was the only means my mother had to get attention. Her throat was one of the few organs that hadn't failed her yet.

"Why does a seventeen-year-old need a king-size bed?!!!"

It's not important!!! You can't walk!!!

"We should check into the hotel," Nancy pleaded, tapping the part of her wrist that would support her watch, if she wore one.

"Oh, yeah," I said. "We'd better get going."

Down the hall from my mother's bedroom there's an original Peanuts cartoon from 1962 that encapsulates her world.

Panel one:
Charlie Brown says to Lucy: "It says here that the force of gravitation is 13% less today than it was 4 ½ billion years ago."

Panel two:
Lucy: "Whose fault is that?"
Charlie Brown: "Whose fault is it? It's nobody's fault."

Panel three:
Lucy: "What do you mean nobody's fault! It HAS to be somebody's fault! Somebody's got to take the blame!"

Panel four:
Lucy (with her mouth open really really wide): "FIND A SCAPEGOAT!!"

This was hung back in the day when my mother saw the humor in things.

DAY TWO

I got up extra early and let Nancy sleep in. It was four in the morning our time but I wanted to get this Zoloft intervention over with. As I sat across from my mother while she lay in bed, she reached over and rang her buzzer to call my father.

"What's the matter?"

"I ne-ed this bag of ice re-moved from my le-gs!"

"Why did you ring the buzzer? I can do that."

"Your fa-ther is just stuff-fing his face in the kitch-en and he's three se-conds away!"

"I'm ONE SECOND away!!!"

Until recently, it was believed that our personalities were relatively fixed by the time we reached adulthood. But new research has shown that the neural networks in our brains are in a continual state of flux, which is called neuroplasticity. My mother's neuroplasticity is definitely in flux, and not in a good way.

"Mom. I just wanted to tell you that I've been on Zoloft for the past couple of years and it's really helped me."

"I don't ne-ed it! I am not de-pressed!"

"I'm not depressed either. It's not just for depression. It'll take a little of your edge off. Believe me, it's changed my life."

"I am *not* tak-ing Zo-loft!"

I guess the Ayurveda talk was on hold.

"Why not? It's nothing to be ashamed about."

A year prior to this conversation, during a different hospital visit, my father had signed a consent form and the doctors had smuggled some Paxil into my mom's pile of pills. For five days she had no idea she was on a mood elevator. For five days the medical staff was able to tolerate her. The link was indisputable. Then she discovered that she was unwittingly taking something and stopped. Which I'm still perplexed over. She was refusing to swallow a pill that made her feel better? Why? I mean, one thing my mother's not shy about is taking medication. The previous afternoon I had picked up Percocet, erythromycin and Coumadin from the pharmacy. She also regularly takes Atenolol, Synthroid, Ambien, Lanoxin and Zetia. And those are only the ones I can remember. Was she doing this to spite everyone? Was there any logic to her reluctance?

She rang her buzzer again and screamed for my father.

"This is insane. I can take that bag of ice off your leg, Mom."

"I do not want you to take this bag of ice off of me. Your fath-er can come in here and do it!"

It was hard not to hate her.

I know these are harsh words. But I'm running out of sympathy. I'm running out of patience. She's long run out of excuses for her abusive behavior. She would never have the perfect life, but she could certainly have a much better one. It would do her a lot of good to sit outside and watch a bird catch a fish in the lake. It would do her a lot of good to say hi to a neighbor instead of bitching about them. It would do her a lot of good to do anything, except what she was doing.

My brother-in-law is going blind. He's just a couple of years older than I am and he's going blind. Now, when you receive that information over the phone it doesn't register. Maybe it's an exaggeration. Maybe it's happening really slowly. Well, Nancy and I went out to lunch with him and let me tell you, my brother-in-law is going blind. He couldn't even make it to the bathroom without help. I mention this not to add another layer of benevolence to Debbie. I mention this because my brother-in-law has an amazing attitude. Although he'll probably never be able to see a computer screen for the rest of his life, his outlook is so positive, I'm not at all worried about him. He's already accepted his situation. Thirty-some years after her diagnosis, my mother still hasn't accepted hers.

That night Nancy cooked brisket for my parents and my mother actually came out of her room and sat at the table with us, a miracle in itself. The only other time she'd emerge from her confines was during Knicks games. Her illness had given her a surplus of idle time and my father had turned her on to the world of pro basketball. They'd put on Knicks hats and sweatshirts and watch the MSG channel together in pseudo peace, as if it were a tacit cease-fire. Since I was an ardent Nets fan, my mother would also watch their games, to give us an extra subject to discuss. But as bad as the Knicks had been of late, my mother was worse.

While the potatoes were being warmed up, Nancy and I managed to coerce my father into drinking some wine we had bought (with sulfites). My mother refused. It might interfere with her griping.

"And yo-ur sis-ter in-sists on clean-ing my bath-room! I do not want my bath-room clean-ed!"

Nancy and I gave each other a look, as if to say, "Jesus Christ! *Of course* you want your bathroom cleaned! Shut up already!" Subjects that should have been immune from criticism were dwindling.

Despite the cascade of complaints my father was bubbly and happy, and because he probably hadn't had a drink in twenty years, perhaps a little buzzed.

"I feel gooooooooood," he giggled as he waved his hands in the air comically, his Mighty Thor cap perched atop his head. It had been a long time between smiles.

Then my mother tried to thwart his glee. And not in a fun way. In a mean way.

"I can-not stand th-is!"

"I feel gooooooooood," my father repeated, still ecstatic. He wasn't trying to taunt her, either. If anything, he was offering up some happiness, hoping she would choose to soak some of it up, like unconscious Reiki. It didn't happen.

"I am go-ing back to my ro-om! I can-not tol-er-ate this non-sense!"

Despite another sip of wine, the joy was slowly being sucked out of my father. He continued to wave his hands in the air and repeat his new catchphrase, but it was halfhearted now. The Mighty Thor hat housed no superpowers. He had been defeated yet again.

Multiple sclerosis has taken away more than my mother's ability to walk. It has taken away her sense of humor, her patience, her logic, her reasoning and any shred of optimism. Before all the brisket had disappeared from everyone's plate, she disappeared into her room, no happier than when she had last left it.

DAY THREE
Since my father couldn't get away from the house much, I ran a lot of errands for him: picking up prescriptions from various doctors, dropping them off at pharmacies, going food shopping and mailing comic books for him at the post office. He gave me several comics to mail to Canada to be insured for $1,100, which he said would cost approximately $30. I went to the UPS Store and was the only person on line. The owner of the place, a heavyset New Yorker who resembled one of the Ben and Jerry's guys, proceeded to take seventeen minutes (there was a clock above his head) to fumble his way through my transaction, finally arriving at the monstrous price of $76 to Ottawa. When I questioned the amount and said that my dad was a veteran of mailing things and was familiar with the rates, he told me that was the cheapest he could do. So I paid and went back to my parents' house to see what other errands I needed to run. I handed my father the receipt; he was furious.

"This is one-day service. It didn't need to get there in one day."

"He didn't offer me any other options."

"That's ridiculous."

I was even more livid than my father. So I called the Ben and Jerry's UPS guy and blasted him over the phone. I told him he was a rip-off artist and pointed out that when I questioned the high price, he never countered with lower-priced options. He was incompetent and unethical and I demanded my money back. When he shouted back, I told him to "fuck off" and then slammed down the Donald Duck phone in the living room. I think that was the first time I said the "f" word in my parents' house.

All the hours of Tai Chi, all the yoga, all the ghee, steamed okra and aloe vera juice, all the scanning, all the laminated quotes, all my time with Kenyon, all the Zoloft—washed away in an instant. I was me again. I had failed.

I went into my mother's bedroom to tell my parents what had happened. Obviously, they already knew. I have a really loud voice. The amazing thing was how happy both of them looked. My mother was jubilant seeing me all riled up. And my dad was ecstatic because my mom was jubilant. It was the one pure moment of closeness the three of us shared the entire visit—actually, in many visits. Then, just as when I first began taking Zoloft, I had a moment of clarity; again I had ascended to the heavens and was watching myself from above, behaving as I knew I should. I took a deep breath and told my parents I didn't care about getting my money back.

The myth in my family has been that anger can control things. In reality, yelling at bank supervisors or UPS clerks or people in Hummers does nothing. And attempting to bully my mother into taking Zoloft is just another way of *me* yelling, by proxy of a Pfizer product. If anger was the only way to make my mother happy, then I needed to find another method. My family needed a new myth. I didn't know what, but it couldn't be any more destructive than the one we'd been using for the past thirty years.

Being ripped off $46 led to this revelation. Bread of Shame.

I'm always quick to point out to Nancy and my siblings that my mother still hasn't accepted her disease, but in some ways I haven't either. Although I've lived alongside her illness, I've never really acknowledged it. Just as my brother has tried to run away from it by going back in time, I've skirted over it by running into the future, trying to outrace it. Ironically, the only member of my family who seems to live in the present is my mother. And she'd be better off anywhere else.

Although we consistently speak on the phone three times a week, I've never really told my mother how sorry I am that she can't walk, that she can't drive, that her central nervous system is broken, that her survival depends upon those around her. I've never expressed true compassion for her condition, I've never expressed how her determination fueled me, how she continued to teach when she was first diagnosed, albeit lying on a couch, and how that inspired me to be persistent, whether in bodybuilding, stand-up or writing. I've never told her how lucky I am to have her as a mother. She never hassled me to get better grades (as long as I was trying), she never hassled me to get a "real job" (as long as I was happy), she never pressured me in any way, pre- or post-MS. This is a woman who never tried to control me. I should stop trying to control her. And, as Eileen from Anger Management said, stop trying to have expectations.

DAY FOUR

On our last day in Florida, I sat in my mother's room and stared at her vast collection of Beanie Babies. There were hundreds of them, neatly pressed against one another on shelves housed in glass, trapped.

I hugged my mother good-bye.

"I'm sorry you've had to go through all this."

"Through what?"

"All these years, I've been blocking out that you've been sick. I mean I talk about it with other people but never really with you. I hope you'll forgive me."

She smiled.

The cab honked to bring us back to the airport. I filled up her glass of water and told her I'd see her in March.

On the way out I passed my father in the kitchen and patted his giant stomach with affection and said good-bye. I contemplated throwing out the half gallon of ice cream in the freezer but realized the decision was his.

19

ENDING

After dropping Nancy and our luggage off at home, I picked up Kenyon and took him up to the dog park for a quick run. On the drive through the hilly roads, it dawned on me: today I was extremely calm, but who knew what tomorrow would bring? Or, for that matter, ten minutes from now. Life and little things will always gnaw at me and I'll never be immune to stress. There is no permanent solution to what ails me, be it pills, doctors or snake-oil salesmen. But I'm up for the battle. I'll continue yoga, Tai Chi, an Ayurvedic diet, some Craniosacral therapy, and yes, 50 mg of Zoloft for the time being. And I'll no longer do anything that makes me more tense, like lifting a dumbbell. I'll also continue to try new, unconventional remedies if I think there's a slim chance that they'll help, no matter what it costs or how far I have to drive. Like an alcoholic, I need to keep working on myself day by day, minute by minute. I need to keep my hyper-chondria in check.

Then, as I pulled into the dog park, I saw him. Both of them, actually. First the collie, then the owner. The two-legged one cowered when he saw me. It was the guy who had given me the finger and challenged me to a fight. It was the guy I had maniacally sprinted across the dog park for, like a wide receiver going deep for a Michael Vick pass, except I wanted to spike his head, not a ball. It was the guy who, had I had Marty Feldman's eyes, I would have actually been cornea-to-cornea with. It was the guy who first made me aware, accidentally, that medicine would only take me so far. It was the guy who made me realize I needed to hurry up and get calm. Before my

Zoloft didn't work anymore. Before nothing in my body worked anymore. Before I was dead.

I was probably the last guy in the world he expected to see. After all, when I had chased him to the dog park, I didn't have a dog. Now, well over a year after our "incident," we were reunited.

Personally, I could deal with the tension. Besides, as tense as it was, it was only a fraction of what it was like being near my mother. But I'd had enough needless stress. I walked across the grassy field toward the collie owner, and despite the abundance of witnesses nearby he looked terrified. If he'd had Mace on him, he probably would have emptied the entire canister on me. I was about three feet from him and I smiled.

"Hey!" I said.

"What?" His voice trembled.

"I just wanna say I'm sorry. I'm sorry for what happened. I overreacted. I'm sorry."

I extended my hand for him to shake. After another awkward moment, he shook it. He had a pretty good grip. He probably could've kicked my ass.

I think I'm getting better.

Then, to celebrate, I threw a nearby tennis ball really far for Kenyon. And I tore the radial nerve in my shoulder.

ACKNOWLEDGING

My literary agent, Farley Chase. Without your guidance, encouragement and patience, this book wouldn't be a book.

The innate wisdom of my editor, Peter Borland, who couldn't have been nicer and easier to work with. (Sorry for ending on a preposition, Peter.)

Craig Anton, Jeanine Cornillot, Katherine Eckert, Stan Evans, Rob Forman, Archie Gips, Cynthia Greenburg, Heidi Gutman, Dave Hanson, Lynn Harris, Jonathan Katz, Bonnie Mark, Madeline Martell, Brett Paesel, Sybil Pincus, Rory Rosegarten, Amy Krouse Rosenthal, Rodney Rothman, Mike Royce, Shoe Schuster, Nick Simonds, Grant Taylor and Val Wagner. Thanks for reading, commenting and supporting.

A.J. Jacobs, Peter Griffin and David Granger at *Esquire*. Dana Brown at *Vanity Fair*. Gary Belsky, Neil Janowitz and Brendan O'Connor at *ESPN the Magazine*. Kit Rachlis, Mary Melton and Matt Segal at *Los Angeles*. You're all amazing editors whom I hope to work for until I'm dead.

Harley Tat for hiring me to write thought-bubbles at *Blind Date*. And then—more important—for hiring Nancy a year later or we never would've met.

The world's best yoga teacher, Andrea Marcum. Yes, I know by now I should be able to do a headstand without the wall, but I'm still frightened.

All the doctors who have helped me deal with my neuroses and ailments.

My siblings. Even though our homes and personalities are all over the map, it doesn't feel that way.

My parents for a lifetime of unconditional love. I hope you still speak to me.

My beautiful and super-tolerant wife, Nancy, who makes me laugh at things that used to bug the hell out of me. I hope to repay you by continuing to calm down.

I'd also like to thank the person who invented the acknowledgments page. It's saved me a lot of phone calls.

Visit Brian Frazer online at www.hyper-chondriac.com.